Vein Health and Problems in Lockdown and Isolation

Professor Mark S Whiteley

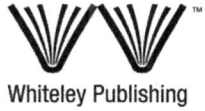

© Whiteley Publishing Ltd. 2020

All rights reserved. No part of this book may be reproduced or transmitted in any form by any means, electronic or mechanical, including photocopying, recording, or by any information storage and retrieval system without written permission of the publisher, except where permitted by law.

Published by Whiteley Publishing Ltd

First paperback edition 2020
ISBN 978-1-908586-10-0

Kindle edition 2020
ISBN 978-1-908586-11-7

This book is sold subject to the condition that it shall not, by way of trade or otherwise, be lent, re-sold, hired out or otherwise circulated in any form of binding or cover other than that in which it is published and without a similar condition including this condition being imposed on the subsequent publisher.

The information in this book has been supplied by the author and has been published by the publisher in good faith.

Contents

Introduction
Vein health and problems in lockdown and isolation

Chapter 1
How can a lockdown or isolation affect vein health?
Page 13

Chapter 2
Symptoms and signs suggesting venous disease
Page 18

Chapter 3
How veins work normally
Page 45

Chapter 4
What can go wrong with veins?
Page 59

Chapter 5
Who is at risk of venous problems during a lockdown or in isolation?
Page 81

Chapter 6
What you can do at home
Page 96

Chapter 7

Treatments for venous conditions and medical versus cosmetic

Page 110

Chapter 8

Covid-19 and venous thrombosis

Page 127

Chapter 9

Keeping your veins healthy and when to look for help

Page 130

Vein health and problems in lockdown and isolation

Professor Mark S Whiteley

Introduction

Our understanding of venous disease has changed massively in the last two decades. The advent of Covid-19 and enforced lockdowns or periods of isolation have helped us concentrate on how such events can impact on venous disease.

The major changes in our understanding of venous disease and treatment have been due to 2 major developments.

Firstly, a new non-invasive test called colour flow venous duplex ultrasound scanning has allowed us to see what is happening inside veins in real time.

Secondly, the development of minimally invasive surgery that can be performed under local anaesthetic in an outpatient clinic has revolutionised venous treatments.

Unfortunately, many doctors have merely replaced their old surgical treatments with the new local anaesthetic minimally invasive treatments, without realising that the understanding of venous disease has changed.

The result of this is that huge numbers of patients get at best misinformed, and at worst the wrong diagnosis and sub-optimal treatments.

Some of the headlines of how venous surgery has changed can be summarised as:

- Varicose veins are not cosmetic and if left untreated, usually deteriorate

- Venous leg ulcers are curable by local anaesthetic surgery, and so most patients do not need long-term compression

- Phlebitis should not be treated with antibiotics and may need anti-coagulation

- Phlebitis can cause pulmonary embolism (clots to the lungs) and all patients should be referred for urgent scans

- Half the patients with venous disease have hidden varicose veins that cannot be identified without a scan, but are prone to deterioration without treatment

- Pelvic varicose veins are the cause of leg varicose veins in 1 in 6 women but are rarely checked or treated

There are a great many other changes in the venous world, but venous diseases do not attract a lot of attention in the medical community. As such they are often treated by a variety of doctors who only treat veins part-time. The public is often led into believing that they are seeing a "vein specialist" because they are called a "vascular surgeon", unaware that most vascular surgeons spend most of their time specialising in arterial surgery which is very different from venous diagnosis and treatment.

Those of us who have dedicated our lives to understanding and treating veins do not currently have an official name, although most of us call ourselves either "venous surgeons" or "phlebologists".

As you will read in this book, venous disease affects more than half of the adult population in one form or another. In addition, the complications of some forms of venous disease can cause chronic ill-health, massive spending by healthcare providers or governments and in some cases can even be fatal.

I wrote this book initially to advise patients on how to look after their veins during a lockdown or isolation period, because of the sudden changes that we have all had to go through during the Covid-19 pandemic. I have been asked to comment in many newspapers and magazines about certain aspects of venous health during this time and have also been contacted by a great many patients with specific questions.

However, as I went through the process of writing this book, I realised that most of the information is relevant to people at other times as well as during a lockdown or during isolation.

Therefore, although I hope that this book is helpful to people who may have had a sudden change of life-style and are at home more than usual, it should also be useful to people who have not been affected during the pandemic. It should also be a useful guide to people once the pandemic is over and we all return to our normal lives.

Mark S Whiteley, November 2020

Chapter 1

How can a lockdown or isolation affect vein health?

The most obvious effect of a lockdown or isolation, and what most people immediately consider, is a change in exercise. In particular, a reduction of exercise throughout the day. People who use personal fitness trackers will be aware of the steps walked when commuting to and from work, around an office, or in activities such as shopping, taking children to and from school, or many of hundreds of other normal daily activities.

Without doubt this is a major factor on vein health. However, it is not only the reduction of exercise, but also the change in the sort of exercise that people have. Although we will go deeper into this later, suffice to say that "veins love walking" and any exercises like walking. Other exercises that burn calories, but do not have the same mechanical mechanisms that walking has, are less useful for vein health.

However, there are other reasons that a lockdown can be detrimental to vein health.

In a lockdown, not only is it likely that people will have changed their diet, but also that they will have changed their pattern of eating and drinking. For instance, there is a lot of evidence from early 2020 that alcohol consumption increased in a significant proportion of people who were in lockdown or isolating.

Although there have not been any clear figures that I have seen on smoking, it is likely that with increased time at home and increased alcohol consumption, smoking is likely to have increased as well. Although the effects of smoking are generally considered to be on the heart and arteries, cigarette smoke also is detrimental to healthy venous biology.

During a lockdown or in isolation, people have more time to read or to browse the Internet. The massive increase in people watching certain videos on the Internet and using online shopping is testimony to the increased use of the World Wide Web. Unfortunately, a lot of the information regarding vein health that is produced commercially is highly suspect and quite often, erroneous.

However, with increased browsing time, people are more subjected to such advertising or false information. It is unfortunately true that people will be more attracted to "miracle cures" or cheap treatments promising fantastic results, than reading scientific literature and seeking proven and audited treatments that appear to take much longer and are more expensive - even though these are actually the treatments that address the problem and work in the medium and long-term!

Increased time spent browsing the Internet is also fuelled by an increase in anxiety that is well documented in many areas of the population during a lockdown. Anxiety about Covid-19 spills over to a general anxiety about health and indeed other areas of life. Being stuck at home and without as many outside distractions of normal life as usual, these concerns can end up playing on the mind. In some, this results in a diagnosable mental health issue. However, in many more, there is just an increased level of anxiety and worry about health generally.

On the positive side, the extra time at home and the increased interest in health has also resulted in many patients who do have venous disease noticing it for the first time. Because venous disease is usually a slowly developing problem, many people do not recognise the early symptoms and signs of varicose veins or hidden varicose veins, and the onset of early complications that can be associated with these.

In a busy life, these can be missed or ignored. Sometimes this can result in patients presenting quite late in the progression of the disease process. One of the advantages of lockdown or isolation in some patients, has been that they have recognised their venous disease at quite an early stage. This has allowed them to seek treatment before significant deterioration or complications have arisen.

In the next chapter we are going to start looking at the symptoms and signs of venous disease. This is to help you recognise possible venous disease and to have an indication as to the severity of any disease present. However, before we do that, it is sensible to have an idea of how many people in the population are affected by venous disease.

One quick note here for the purists. I am using the term "venous disease" as this is a widely accepted and understood term. Many in the venous world dislike the term "disease" for venous conditions and prefer the term "venous disorders". For the simple understanding of this book, the terms "venous disease" and "venous disorders" are interchangeable.

How many people are affected by venous disease?

Although we will discuss the different forms of venous disease later in this book, the commonest sort of venous disease is varicose veins.

We all use the words varicose veins, but this isn't a very good term. When we say "varicose veins" we are using a description of something that can be seen clinically. When someone stands, and veins bulge abnormally on the legs, or around the buttocks or intimate areas, we call these varicose veins.

Population studies have shown that when this simple definition of varicose veins is used, approximately 15-20% of the adult population have these visible varicose veins.

However, as we will find out later, these visible bulging veins are not the problem. These veins merely bulge and become prominent because some of the underlying veins are not working properly. This malfunctioning allows blood to flow the wrong way down the affected veins. The reversal of normal flow is called "venous reflux".

Venous reflux can either be passive due to gravity, or active due to muscle pumping. Whichever way venous reflux occurs, it can allow the abnormal blood flow to fill and stretch veins near the surface. Hence the presence of varicose veins actually shows the presence of venous reflux in underlying veins.

This is an important distinction. For every person with visible varicose veins, it is estimated that there is another who has the same venous reflux in the leg or pelvic veins, but who do not have any visible varicose veins bulging on the surface.

Of course, if the bulging varicose veins were the problem, then this underlying hidden reflux would not matter. The problem is that it is the venous reflux that causes most of the problems in venous disease. We will discuss this fully later, but for the present time it is important to note that it is the venous reflux that causes most of the problems, not the visible bulging veins.

Medically, this abnormal venous reflux has got several different names such as "superficial venous incompetence" (SVI) or "superficial venous reflux" (SVR) or "chronic venous incompetence" (CVI) as well as several other different variations. In 2009 I started using the term "hidden varicose veins" on my websites to try to help simplify this condition and make it more understandable. Then in 2011 I published the term in a book called "**Understanding Venous Reflux - the cause of varicose veins and venous leg ulcers**". I am delighted to find that the name "hidden varicose veins" has now become quite widespread in the medical literature.

Population studies have shown that approximately 15-20% of the adult population have hidden varicose veins. In other words, they have the same venous reflux as the patients with visible varicose veins, but do not have the outward signs of bulging veins.

Putting all of this together and understanding that it is the venous reflux that causes most of the problems in venous disease, it is clear that approximately 30-40% of the adult population has venous reflux in leg veins whether they are visible or not. The development of symptoms and/or signs that are recognised as venous disease, or complications that are seen to be due to venous disease, is merely a factor of how quickly the condition deteriorates in each individual person. Many of the factors that determine this will be discussed later in the book.

There are other causes of venous disease including stasis (blood not moving much in the veins) and obstruction (when blood flow through the veins is impeded) and these can present with a host of different conditions.

Although we will concentrate on leg veins in this book, it is important to remember the pelvic veins. All venous blood leaving the legs must flow up the pelvic veins. As with all veins, these can also go wrong and allow venous reflux.

Pelvic vein reflux has become a major area of research and development of new investigations and treatment. Not only does reflux from the pelvic veins affect leg veins, it is also the cause of several other conditions. These are pelvic congestion syndrome, vaginal varicose veins, and varicocele (varicose veins around the testicle). It is also implicated in haemorrhoids (piles) and some cases of erectile dysfunction.

The rest of this book will start explaining the above in more detail. However, it is important to note at this stage that approximately one third of adults have venous reflux in their leg veins. As this is the commonest underlying cause of venous disease, this equates to a very large number of people affected in the population.

Chapter 2

Symptoms and signs suggesting venous disease

In medicine, patients suffer from symptoms. These are the things that you feel when you have a certain condition or illness. Doctors then look for signs, which are visible or palpable changes that suggest or confirm a certain condition.

Although, as we will discuss later, the underlying cause of venous disease comes down to relatively simple changes in the function of normal veins, the different ways venous disease is felt by the patient or can be seen by the patient or their doctor are quite varied.

They vary in significance and severity. Once I have listed the different symptoms and signs, I will go into each in more detail.

In medicine, doctors like to classify and order diseases and disease processes. Although this is helpful for doctors who see hundreds or thousands of patients with similar conditions, it is not much help for a person who is trying to assess whether they have venous disease, and, if so, how serious it may be.

Therefore, I have listed the commonest symptoms and signs of venous disease below. Although most patients with significant venous disease will have one of the following, it is quite possible to have more than one:

- Aching, heavy or tired leg or legs

- Thread veins/spider veins on leg or ankle

- Profuse green veins over the leg or legs that may be associated with thread veins or not

- Bulging veins (varicose veins)

- Swelling of part or all of the lower limb

- Eczema of the lower leg just above the ankle
- Red or brown skin changes around the ankle
- Hard shiny skin just above the ankle
- Sudden appearance of tender lumps of the leg or legs that may be colourless or red
- An open sore on the lower leg or foot (called an ulcer)
- Profuse bleeding of dark blood from a bulging vein on the leg or foot

Symptoms and signs that might be due to venous disease but also might be due to other causes:

- Swelling of the leg but particularly of the toes, on one or both sides
- Swelling of both legs exactly the same on each side
- A patch of hot red skin that looks inflamed and increases in size, often causing a temperature and feeling unwell

I will now go through each of these in turn.

Aching, heavy or tired leg or legs

Varicose veins or hidden varicose veins rarely cause considerable pain. The discomfort that most people get with varicose veins or hidden varicose veins is an aching, or a feeling that the legs are just heavy or tired. Sometimes it is described as a "throbbing".

These symptoms tend to get worse during the day as most people are on their legs throughout the day. Usually the symptoms are best first thing in the morning having had a whole night in bed. We will come on to discuss the way that venous reflux causes inflammation in the legs later, but most people will have an understanding that gravity plays a part. As such, the longer you are sitting or standing with your legs down, the more the legs are likely to ache.

Obviously, these sorts of symptoms can be improved with elevating the legs, particularly when they are elevated higher than the heart. Many patients with varicose veins or hidden varicose veins volunteer that when they come home after a day at work, they lie on their backs with their legs propped up against a wall. This brings considerable relief.

In addition, medical support stockings also help in a good proportion of patients with this problem.

Interestingly, some patients find the discomfort worse when they first get into bed. This may seem strange as the legs are elevated when in bed, but it is a clear symptom in some patients. The usual reason appears to be that when patients are up and about, they ignore the aching in their legs. When they get into bed, and try to relax, all the other distractions disappear allowing the discomfort to become more obvious.

In addition, there is a process called "accommodation". Many people will wear an uncomfortable garment such as an itchy shirt all day. During the day they get used to it and ignore it. However, when they take the garment off at the end of the day, they suddenly feel the discomfort all over again even though it has been removed. This is because the body is sometimes better at feeling changes than feeling the same chronic discomfort that does not change over a long time. This acceptance of a discomfort is called "accommodation".

Finally, in this section, it is worth emphasising that varicose veins or hidden varicose veins rarely cause actual pain. Venous discomfort is much more of a chronic low-level ache, hence the often-used terms of aching, heavy or tired legs. If there is severe pain, this is almost always due to a sudden change and increased inflammation.

Examples of such sudden changes are the formation of a clot in a vein such as a superficial venous thrombus (commonly called "phlebitis"), or a deep vein thrombosis (DVT), an acute infection such as cellulitis or some other non-venous cause. These will all be discussed later.

It is interesting that in the past, many patients have been put off having their varicose veins treated "because they are not painful". Over the years, doctors, insurance companies and other bodies who fund healthcare have managed to put patients off having treatment for varicose veins by asking "are they painful?"

When the patient says "no", it appears logical that if they don't hurt, they are not severe enough to need treatment.

This is complete nonsense.

There are a great many medical conditions that need treatment but do not cause pain. For instance, if you have a cataract, the reason you get treatment is so you can see again. If you had to wait for it to become painful, you would never have it treated. Other conditions such as aortic aneurysm or breast cancer do not usually cause pain but need treatment to prevent rupture in the former case and spread in the latter case.

Similarly, the deterioration of venous disease from varicose veins to swollen ankles, skin damage, leg ulcers, bleeding or the formation of clots is rarely painful, and the reason to treat the veins early is to prevent such deterioration. It is not to take away pain. Therefore, linking pain to the need to operate on varicose veins appears to have arisen solely to persuade patients that their varicose veins do not need treatment!

Thread veins/spider veins on leg or ankle

Small red, purple or blue veins or networks of veins particularly on the legs are often called "thread veins", "spider veins", "broken capillaries" or other similar terms. Medically they are called "telangiectasia".

Although obvious to see in many people, the problem with these sorts of veins is that they are very common. Although they can point to underlying venous disease, they can also exist without any underlying problem.

Research from the Edinburgh Vein Study published in 2008 by Prof CV Ruckley and his team showed that thread veins (telangiectasia) are very common in both adult men and adult women. Indeed, they noted that on the right leg 79% of men and 88% of women showed telangiectasia.

Therefore, it can be thought that telangiectasia are so common, they do not help us in determining who might have more severe underlying venous disease. However, there is more to it than that.

Firstly, there appears to be a link between telangiectasia and underlying venous reflux. Not everybody with thread veins has underlying reflux, but it does increase the chance. Indeed, with very careful scanning, almost 9 out of every 10 patients with telangiectasia have some venous reflux feeding them and approximately 40% will have major venous reflux. On top of this, approximately 15% of these thread veins will be fed by incompetent perforating veins.

As such, patients with significant thread veins (telangiectasia) are more likely to have underlying hidden varicose veins, even if no bulging varicose veins are seen on the surface.

Another thing to note with thread veins or telangiectasia of the legs is their distribution. Some of these are typical but not of great concern. For instance, many women will show thread veins on their outer thighs, often related to venous reflux in a feeding vein arising from below, at the level of the knee. Although not clinically significant, these sort of thread veins are only treated successfully if the underlying feeding veins are treated as well.

On the other hand, thread veins that are seen as an inverted blue "fan", radiating downwards and away from the inner ankle joint and onto the foot, is often a sign of significant venous disease. These profuse and dark thread veins under the inner ankle joint are called "phlebectasia corona". In the past, these were thought to be a sign of a previous deep-vein thrombosis (DVT). However, it has now become apparent that it is more usual that they are associated with hidden varicose veins.

Therefore, patients with this pattern of thread veins around the ankle, potentially have significant hidden varicose veins. Therefore, they are likely to have more significant venous disease than just cosmetic thread veins.

It is for this reason that any venous specialist would always insist on a full colour flow duplex ultrasound scan of the leg veins before ever considering starting any treatment on leg thread veins.

Profuse green veins over the legs that may be associated with thread veins or not

Visible green veins on the legs, that do not bulge, are called "reticular veins". They are quite commonly found in slim people without much body fat.

Although they can be distressing cosmetically, they are rarely a source of concern by themselves.

They can be associated with underlying venous reflux or hidden varicose veins, and therefore much of what has been written about thread veins above is appropriate to these veins as well. They can be treated cosmetically by sclerotherapy, but should only ever be treated after a venous duplex ultrasound scan has excluded an underlying venous problem.

Of course, similarly with thread veins, the presence of profuse reticular veins and other symptoms or signs of venous disease would increase the chances of a significant underlying venous problem.

In addition, profuse reticular veins on one leg and not the other would significantly increase the chance of an underlying venous problem on the affected side.

Bulging veins (varicose veins)

- Legs

The most obvious and most widely known venous problem is varicose veins. In reality, and as discussed previously, this term merely means abnormally dilated or enlarged veins, that are visible on standing.

We will get into a better understanding of varicose veins later on in this book, but at the present time it is useful to know a few things about them.

Firstly, varicose veins of the legs are usually caused by only one of the causes of venous disease - venous reflux. In the past, venous reflux was thought to be simple. Unfortunately, most doctors who treat varicose veins are still under this misapprehension. According to this simple view, there are two main veins in the legs that can cause varicose veins. The first is the great saphenous vein, and the second is the small saphenous vein. Before 2001 these were called the "long saphenous vein" and the "short saphenous vein". Amazingly I still see reports from doctors who treat veins, still using these outdated terms. It shows that these doctors have not read any contemporary venous research nor been to any venous meetings of note for two decades!

Over the last 20 years, considerable research performed by my team at The Whiteley Clinic has shown that varicose veins can be caused by reflux in any one or more of 150 different veins per leg. These might be long veins such as the saphenous veins, small veins perforating through the muscle called incompetent perforating veins, or veins coming out of the pelvis and passing into the legs. It is not surprising that so many people get their varicose veins back again after treatment by doctors who only recognise and treat the great and small saphenous veins.

Varicose veins due to venous reflux will slowly deteriorate with time. The deterioration is actually due to the venous reflux rather than the varicose veins themselves. As we have already noted, the bulging varicose veins are just a sign of the venous reflux. The general deterioration is from visible varicose veins to visible varicose veins with aching, tired or heavy legs.

The next stage is then swelling of the ankle. If the venous reflux has not been treated by this stage, the next stage is then eczema, red stains or brown stains around the lower leg just above the ankle joint. In some people this can result in a hard shiny area called "lipodermatosclerosis" (LDS). If this gets very tight around the lower leg and the calf bulges it can form a classic inverted "champagne bottle" leg. If the skin breaks down, an open sore called a venous ulcer can appear.

It is important to note that this is not a stepwise progression and some people will progress directly to one of the later stages without necessarily going through previous stages. Indeed, many patients will progress to brown stains of the skin or a venous leg ulcer, without even seeing a bulging varicose vein at all - the "hidden varicose veins" that I have spoken about previously.

It is interesting that we have found that some patients with visible varicose veins found that their varicose veins became painful during lockdown, despite not having noticed the pain beforehand. This may be due to different levels of exercise during lockdown or might represent the extra time people have had to consider themselves and their health as discussed previously. Whatever the cause, we have seen a significant number of people who have known that they have leg varicose veins but have not previously had any symptoms at all, but have become quite distressed by the tiredness of their legs and aching within weeks of starting lockdown.

With regards varicose veins and pain, we have already discussed that varicose veins are rarely associated with any significant pain and usually only cause aching, heavy or tired legs. Any severe pain is almost always due to another condition such as clot, infection or some other disease process.

Having said this, there are some areas where varicose veins can cause much more concern. Sometimes varicose veins on the legs are only dilated because they are bypassing a blocked deep vein. Patients with this usually have other problems such as a previous history of deep vein thrombosis or trauma/surgery to the leg. In addition, this leg will often be more swollen than the other leg. There may well be skin discolouration on this side or even brown stains.

Sometimes, varicose veins can be present in a patient with a large birthmark on the thigh or buttock area. In such patients, the leg is often larger on this side and sometimes longer. These changes are not acute and have almost always been visible since birth. Such patients have a condition called Klippel Trenaunay syndrome (KTS). In the past such patients have been told they cannot be treated successfully and so are destined to a life of compression stockings. However, at The Whiteley Clinic we have been treating increasing numbers of such patients successfully using combinations of specialised treatments. However, this is a very specialised subject and further discussion of this is beyond the scope of this book.

Varicose veins can occur elsewhere, and these can indicate different conditions.

- Vulva, vagina, scrotum, buttocks, anus

Varicose veins around the vagina and vulva indicate pelvic varicose veins, a condition called pelvic congestion syndrome (PCS). This is relatively common and can cause one or more symptoms such as aching in the pelvis with a dragging sensation on standing or sitting, irritable bowel syndrome, irritable bladder, deep pain on sexual intercourse or after sexual intercourse (deep dyspareunia), low back pain or hip pain. Unfortunately, most gynaecologists and family doctors do not recognise this condition and it has been left to venous experts such as myself to do most of the research in this area. As such, it is estimated that 30% (one in three) of women attending gynaecology out-patients with chronic pelvic pain are misdiagnosed as either endometriosis or told there is nothing wrong with them.

Again, although interesting, it is beyond the scope of this book to discuss this subject further as pelvic congestion syndrome is a chronic condition that is unlikely to have an acute deterioration during a lockdown or isolation. It is possible that some women will recognise themselves from this description. Further information can be found in my book "***Pelvic Congestion Syndrome - chronic pelvic pain and pelvic venous disorders***".

Interestingly, haemorrhoids or piles are often pelvic varicose veins with the lower varicose veins bulging from the anus. Traditionally these have been treated by bowel surgeons merely because of where they appear. However, increasingly, venous surgeons are now starting to take an interest in this area as the underlying condition is more likely to be a problem with the pelvic veins than a problem with the bowels. During lockdown or isolation, the most likely emergency related to haemorrhoids is that they either thrombose or bleed.

If they thrombose, this means that the blood inside the haemorrhoid clots. The haemorrhoid will become swollen, hard and exceptionally painful. Depending on the severity and size, you can use painkillers and ice in the short term but if the pain and size is significant, you should contact your family doctor or emergency department as a matter of some urgency.

Bleeding haemorrhoids should also be treated as a medical emergency. It is rare that the bleeding is sufficient to be life-threatening but if it becomes profuse, you may need urgent admission to your local emergency department. In addition, it is possible that you have haemorrhoids, but the bleeding is actually coming from another source inside the bowel.

- Abdomen

Varicose veins running over the pubic bone, either under or just over the pubic hair, is a very worrying sign. Such veins appear when one of the major veins in the pelvis becomes blocked, and venous blood tries to bypass the blockage by dilating these veins on the surface.

Veins such as these appear as a long-term response to a blockage and rarely occur suddenly. Nowadays the underlying blocked veins can often be reopened with a stent. However, it is uncommon that this sort of vein will suddenly appear without there being other symptoms and signs, such as a very swollen and painful leg on one side. We will discuss these other symptoms and signs later. If you did notice this sort of vein, it is worth investigating but not necessarily as an urgent case unless you have any other symptoms or signs.

It is also possible to get varicose veins running up both flanks, on the sides of the abdomen. This happens when the deep veins in the pelvis and abdomen get blocked. Just as with varicose veins over the pubic area, this rarely happens in the short-term without other very major changes. Again, it can be treated nowadays by opening the deeper veins in a large proportion of cases. However, unless there is some other problem, it is not an acute condition that needs urgent care.

Varicose veins radiating away from the belly button (umbilicus) is a condition called "Caput Medusae" or the "Medusa's head" after the Greek mythological woman who had snakes for hair. When this is present, it is almost always due to liver disease and nothing to do with venous disease. If you did notice this, you would certainly need to speak to your doctor but would not need to see a venous surgeon.

- Chest, arms, hands, breasts, face

Any varicose veins above the level of the heart or on the arms, are not due to gravity or venous reflux. Some of these are merely cosmetic. At The Whiteley Clinic we are now developing many treatments to take away non-tender veins on the face, breasts, arms and hands that patients do not like the look of.

However, large varicose veins that appear over the shoulder or neck on one side only, usually indicates there is a blocked vein in the armpit. This is not usually an acute event, unless there is a sudden swelling of the arm with associated pain, which would entail an urgent visit to the emergency department.

Swelling of part or all of the lower limb

Swelling of part, or all, of a lower limb can be a source of great concern. There are a number of different causes of leg swelling, some completely benign and others that are more serious. Therefore, we need to consider certain aspects of the swelling and any associated symptoms to help us make a decision as to what to do.

Such considerations might be anatomical (both legs or just one leg), speed of onset of swelling, severity of swelling both in terms of size and whether the skin has become very tight, any discolouration and any associated pain. If the leg swelling has been present for some time, it is important to know whether the swelling stops at the ankle and upper foot, or whether the toes are significantly swollen as well.

Probably the first thing to consider is whether the swelling affects one leg or both. If both legs are swelling to the same extent, then it is much more likely that the swelling is due to a generalised condition. Such generalised conditions can be low protein levels, heart failure with fluid retention, certain medications, or other medical conditions. It is possible for there to be symmetrical venous disease causing such swelling, although this is less likely.

If one leg is swollen and the other not, or significantly less, then venous disease is more likely. Alternatively, lymphoedema can also affect one side alone.

The next thing to consider is the speed of onset of the swelling. If the leg or legs swell slowly throughout the day, and this has been going on for some time, then this is much less likely to be an acute problem. A slow swelling of both legs that is symmetrical is likely to be a generalised medical condition. One leg swelling slowly alone throughout the day, or more than the other side, can be due to venous disease or lymphatic disease. The difference between the two is usually that venous swelling usually stops around the ankle whereas in lymphoedema, the swelling goes right down and includes the toes.

Of much more concern is if one leg swells suddenly, having never had a swelling problem before. When this happens, we start worrying about deep vein thrombosis (DVT).

A smaller DVT of the calf or lower leg will often cause some swelling of the ankle, often with discomfort in the calf muscle such as aching. Standing upright with the foot flat on the ground causes pain in the calf as the calf muscle is stretched. The clot causes inflammation in the veins. As these veins are deep within the calf muscle, this stretching of the calf muscle is painful. Medically this is called the "Homan's sign". Generally, 50% of people who have this sort of clear history of a calf DVT will have a calf DVT. The other 50% will have some other condition mimicking it such as a ruptured Bakers cyst.

A Bakers cyst is an "out-pouching" of the membranes and fluid of the knee joint behind the knee. This area is known medically as the "popliteal fossa". The pouch of joint fluid (called "synovial fluid") that usually lubricates the knee joint can bulge into this space. If it ruptures, the thick synovial fluid flows into the calf muscle. This is very irritating, and the calf muscle becomes inflamed and tender. This gives the swelling, tenderness and pain on extension that mimics a calf DVT.

The only clear way to tell between the two is to have a colour flow duplex ultrasound scan of the veins. Many hospitals will perform a blood test to look for inflammation called a D-dimer test. If this is positive, the patient is started on anticoagulation and booked in for a scan at a later date. Specialist vein clinics will tend to go straight for a colour flow duplex ultrasound scan. Some hospitals will still perform venography injecting contrast into the veins and using x-rays to look for blocked veins. However, this test is now quite dated.

What is clear from this description is that if a below knee DVT is suspected, you should seek medical help immediately. This is not something that should be left undiagnosed or untreated as a thrombosis in the deep veins can extend, getting larger and potentially affecting more veins up the leg. Uncommonly for a calf DVT, but still possible, is some of the clot flying off through the veins to the lungs, a condition called pulmonary embolism.

Moving to another possible scenario, if one leg swells suddenly and massively, affecting the thigh as well as the calf, then this is highly likely to be a large DVT in the thigh vein or even pelvic vein. If this happens acutely, the leg will feel very tight and will ache severely. The pain can be intense. This is a medical emergency and you need to seek help immediately. You should call for an ambulance and attend an emergency department.

In the most severe cases, the leg can swell suddenly, be painful and go either blue or white. In this sort of case, you will not be left in any doubt about the swelling, pain nor skin colour change. The swelling is massive and affects the whole leg up to the groin. The skin is very tight and painful.

These are rare conditions but if they happen, once again it is an emergency. These conditions are called "phlegmasia cerulea dolens" (which basically means a painful blue leg - phlegmasia = inflammation, cerulea = blue, dolens = painful) or "phlegmasia alba dolens" (the same but white rather than blue). Both of these conditions only occur in people who are very sick with other problems. If this happens, you need to get straight into hospital for full investigations and treatment, not only of the leg but to look for why it happened.

Eczema of the lower leg just above the ankle

Eczema is an inflammation of the skin that causes the skin to go red, dry and flaky. It is also usually intensely itchy. Some people who have multiple allergies (medically called "atopic") can develop eczema anywhere on their body. Eczema is also related to stress and worsens at such times.

Many people who do not usually suffer from eczema can develop eczema in areas where their skin gets inflamed. For instance, eczema might develop on the scalp if a new shampoo is used that doesn't agree with them or might appear on the hands and wrists if a new washing up detergent is used. These are examples where the person in question does not normally get eczema but whose skin only needs a little push to react to something that irritates it.

Inflammation around the ankle from varicose veins or hidden varicose veins can push the skin into developing eczema in the local area.

Interestingly, most skin reactions to varicose veins or hidden varicose veins occur in an area on the inner aspect of the leg, above the ankle bone but below the calf muscle. This is called the "gaiter" area as it is the area covered by a bishop's gaiter.

Although this is the commonest place for venous eczema to occur, other areas of skin on the leg can be inflamed due to varicose veins or hidden varicose veins. Hence the same venous eczema can occur on the lower leg on the outer aspect rather than the inner aspect, or sometimes over the actual bulging varicose veins themselves even if this is above the knee.

One of the easiest ways to determine whether eczema on the legs is due to varicose veins (hidden or otherwise) or is just part of a general eczema is to see whether there is eczema elsewhere on the body at the same time. If you have eczema on one of your legs, but also have eczema on one of your arms and in your hair at the same time, it is much less likely to be due to varicose veins or hidden varicose veins. If, however, all of your eczema is on one leg or both legs, and particularly if you can see varicose veins, then venous eczema is more likely.

The only effective way of treating venous eczema is to have the underlying venous reflux treated, getting rid of the varicose veins or hidden varicose veins. Traditional treatments of emollients, steroid creams or support stockings are not treatments of venous eczema but are only treatments of skin eczema.

As venous eczema is caused by a reaction of the skin to the underlying venous reflux in varicose veins or hidden varicose veins, leaving the veins untreated means that no treatment put on the skin will have any long-term effect at all. As such skin treatments are effectively useless in venous eczema. Indeed, steroids can actually damage the skin and should not be used unless for quick symptomatic relief before the veins are treated properly.

If venous eczema does occur during lockdown or isolation, this isn't an emergency that needs treatment straight away. However, an appointment should be made with a venous expert as soon as the lockdown finishes to investigate the underlying venous reflux and to arrange treatment. Symptomatic relief with emollients, steroid cream and/or compression stockings and even antihistamines may help to reduce any symptoms of itching until lockdown or isolation has finished.

If the rules of your lockdown do allow you to attend medical appointments, then venous eczema is one of the medical conditions that would allow you to attend a medical appointment for diagnosis and treatment, to prevent further deterioration.

Red or brown skin changes around the ankle

Inflammation around the lower leg from venous disease can cause red staining or brown staining (haemosiderin). The redness is from inflammation. The brown stain is from chronic inflammation resulting in some of the blood in the skin capillaries breaking down, releasing the iron into the skin. Iron is toxic to the skin and so is surrounded by a pigment called haemosiderin. This is a brown colour. The longer the inflammation has been present, the less redness and the more brown staining is present.

The usual site of the staining is the "gaiter" area as described above. This is the area above the inner ankle bone (called the medial malleolus) but below the calf muscle. However, sometimes these stains can be found around the ankle joint, or even below this point and on to the inner aspect of the foot and heel. In addition, in some patients this red or brown stain can be found on the front of the shin or on the outside of the lower leg between the outside ankle bone (called the lateral malleolus) and the calf muscle.

These inflammatory skin changes can be due to varicose veins or hidden varicose veins and can be present without any other signs or symptoms of venous disease. Sometimes they can be associated with some swelling of the ankle. This swelling tends to be less severe in patients with venous reflux due to varicose veins or hidden varicose veins compared to other causes of leg swelling.

If there is additional obstruction or stasis (see later for description of these other conditions) then they can be quite significant swelling of the ankle associated with these red or brown stains.

It is highly unlikely that these red or brown stains will occur acutely over a few days during lockdown or isolation. They tend to slowly increase over many weeks and months, being seen to worsen over the years.

Therefore, although they are important signs of venous disease, and indicate that you need to see a venous specialist, red or brown stains are not signs of an urgent problem in themselves. Hence the appearance of red stains or brown stains around your ankles during lockdown or isolation, usually mean that you have only just noticed something that has been developing over time.

Provided there are no other symptoms or signs, you just need to book an appointment with a venous specialist for a colour flow duplex ultrasound scan and assessment once lockdown or your isolation is finished. This will allow you to plan treatment and to reverse the deterioration, in order to prevent leg ulceration or other complications.

If the rules of your lockdown do allow you to attend medical appointments, then red or brown stains as described here are medical conditions that would allow you to attend a medical appointment for diagnosis and treatment, to prevent further deterioration.

If you have red or brown stains around the ankle that have been there for some time, but suddenly get swelling of the leg, then please follow the advice of the swelling of the leg section rather than this section relating to the long-term colour change.

Hard shiny skin just above the ankle

In some patients, the same inflammation from venous disease that occurs in the lower leg causing the red or brown stains as seen in the previous section, or even the venous eczema as seen previously, can cause a hardening of the skin and underlying tissues. In these patients, the skin often becomes smooth and shiny and sometimes also discoloured.

This is called lipodermatosclerosis (LDS). Breaking this name down in medical terms, lipo = fat, dermato = skin, sclerosis = hardening. Hence lipodermatosclerosis means a hardening of both the skin and the underlying fat.

Quite often LDS and haemosiderin deposition can occur at the same time. LDS almost always occurs in the gaiter area - between the inner ankle bone (medial malleolus) and the calf muscle of the inner lower leg.

When LDS becomes severe and affects the whole of the lower leg from ankle to calf all around the circumference, then the calf can bulge and the lower leg tighten and narrow. This gives the appearance of an inverted champagne bottle and is called a "champagne bottle leg".

LDS is a chronic condition that takes months and years to form. If you notice this during lockdown or isolation, then it has probably been developing for a long time. It is a clear sign of chronic venous disease that is worsening, and you will need to book an appointment to see a venous specialist to have a consultation and colour flow duplex ultrasound scan after lockdown, with a view to getting treatment and preventing further deterioration and complications. However, there is no acute need to be seen during lockdown or isolation unless the rules of your lockdown allow you to attend medical appointments. If so, then LDS is a medical reason to attend a medical appointment for investigation and treatment, to prevent further deterioration.

Sudden appearance of tender lumps of the legs that may be colourless or red

The sudden appearance of tender lumps on the legs which might be visible or might only be found by touch, is almost always due to "phlebitis".

This is a really important condition that can affect people with varicose veins or hidden varicose veins during lockdown or isolation and needs urgent attention. In addition, the international guidelines (both in the UK and the USA) changed in 2012 and many doctors are not aware of this, putting patients at risk. I will explain this now in this section.

"Phlebitis" basically means "inflammation of a vein" from "phleb" = vein and "itis" = inflammation. In this case, inflammation is caused by a blood clot in the superficial veins just under the skin. As the blood clot inside a vein is called a "thrombus", and the process of a thrombus forming is called "thrombosis", the proper name for this condition is "superficial venous thrombosis". However, some older doctors still call it "superficial venous thrombophlebitis".

The presentation really depends upon whether you have varicose veins or hidden varicose veins before the superficial venous thrombosis develops.

If you have visible varicose veins which one day suddenly go hard, tender, lumpy and frequently the skin covering them turns red, then you will know without a shadow of doubt that you have superficial venous thrombosis (or "phlebitis").

Some people develop superficial venous thrombosis in veins that are not varicose and are not visible on the surface – as in hidden varicose veins. Such people might never have been aware that they had any vein problem at all.

In these patients, the clot that forms and causes inflammation is in a vein that is deeper under the skin. Quite often such lumps can only be felt rather than seen. They will still be tender and usually feel more like a hard "sausage" lying vertically up the leg rather than a simple lump, although this is not always the case. The deeper the vein with the clot in it, the less likely a lump is to be seen on the surface and the less likely there is to be any change of the colour of the overlying skin. However, the thrombosed vein will still be tender, and the lump should be palpable.

In the past, doctors and nurses used to think that a clot in the superficial veins of the legs was not important. It is not a deep vein thrombosis because it is in the superficial veins and therefore was thought to be only a cause of pain. Some doctors who did not understand the condition at all would give antibiotics! As there is no infection this is ridiculous. However, there are some doctors who will always treat anything that is hot, red, painful and swollen with antibiotics as they do not understand there are other causes of inflammation apart from infection!

Slightly more enlightened doctors would use non-steroidal anti-inflammatory drugs such as aspirin or ibuprofen to reduce the inflammation and help with the pain, and also give support stockings for further pain relief.

However, in 2012 there were two major publications from committees reviewing research into thrombosis and blood clots. One was in the USA and one in the UK. Both showed that "phlebitis" (superficial venous thrombosis) was not quite as benign as people had previously thought. Because it is basically a clot in the superficial veins, there are some instances when that clot can move into the deep veins and from there to the lungs.

Therefore everyone with phlebitis should have a colour flow duplex ultrasound scan to check that it is superficial venous thrombosis causing the lumps and tenderness, and then identifying whether it is one of the simple ones that can be treated with non-steroidal anti-inflammatory tablets and stockings, or one of the more serious kinds that requires full anticoagulation (blood thinners) to reduce the risk of a clot to the lungs (pulmonary embolism).

We will discuss this fully later. As far as this section of the book is concerned, it is important that you know that the sudden appearance of tender lumps in the legs, that might be either visible and red, or deeper and therefore only found by touch, may well be phlebitis and that an urgent colour flow duplex ultrasound scan is needed to determine correct treatment. You should not wait until the end of lockdown or isolation and you should seek expert opinion immediately.

An open sore on the lower leg or foot (called an ulcer)

The sudden appearance of an open sore for no obvious reason, or a wound that will not heal, on the lower leg, ankle or foot is usually a venous leg ulcer.

Although some people are aware about ulcers and what they look like, I find a surprising number of my patients are quite shocked when they first realise that they have a leg ulcer.

Firstly, an ulcer can affect adults of any age. As with a lot of myths about varicose veins, there are many misperceptions about venous leg ulcers. The most common is that it only affects very old people. It is certainly true that it is more common the older you get, but I have treated and cured many people in their 30s, 40s and 50s who have had severe venous leg ulcers that have ruined their quality-of-life before I have cured them permanently. Indeed, the youngest patient I have had with a venous leg ulcer was 19 years old.

Secondly, a great number of people do not realise that the non-healing wounds they have is actually a venous leg ulcer! I have lost count of the number of people that I have treated for venous leg ulcers that have told me it cannot be an ulcer because they remember when they first injured the leg. Sometimes they will remember a cat scratching the leg, or a dog bumping into their lower legs. Often, they remember banging their legs against furniture or other objects. For some reason they feel that because they can remember the original injury that broke the skin, this cannot be a leg ulcer.

Of course, it is not the injury that is the problem, but rather the body's response to injury. A normal person with normal venous circulation will only notice the original injury. Many people get scratches, cuts or bangs against their lower legs every day. Usually, the body's normal healing processes cause inflammation in the area, which is part of the healing response. A scab forms on any break in the skin, and the skin heals. We don't usually pay much notice to such small traumas.

However, people who have venous disease such as varicose veins or hidden varicose veins have an abnormal response to injury for reasons we will detail later in this book. This means that there is ongoing chronic inflammation in the lower leg, which is very different from the acute inflammation that happens when a healing process is started. The result of this is that the skin does not heal, and the wound becomes an open sore.

Unfortunately, affected patients, doctors and nurses start concentrating on the open sore or ulcer. This is not surprising as the ulcer is what concerns the patient and it is of course the most obvious thing to see. However, it is the venous disease in the legs that has stopped the skin healing and the ulcer will not heal properly until the venous disease is treated first. We have to get to the cause of the problem rather than just treat the signs seen on the surface.

Many people who get an ulcer on their lower legs during lockdown or isolation will already know that they have varicose veins. Others may have hidden varicose veins and only know that one or both of their legs have been swelling for some time, or they have had red or brown discolouration of the lower legs before the ulcer appeared. Sometimes, patients have previously had deep vein thrombosis and occasionally, there can be more complex causes for ulcers such as artery disease.

We will come to talk about these different sorts of ulcers later in the book. The most important point at this stage is to recognise that an open wound or sore that does not heal quickly and normally is almost definitely a leg ulcer and needs to be treated as such.

For hundreds of years, doctors and nurses have treated leg ulcers with dressings and compression. However, since the 1990s we have known in the scientific world that this is not the optimal treatment, and to get rid of the leg ulcer we need to treat the underlying venous reflux (varicose veins or hidden varicose veins) which is usually the cause.

This was proven in two randomised controlled trials, one in 2007 and one in 2018 and is now without doubt. Indeed, the national guidelines in the UK (NICE clinical guidelines CG 168) which were published in summer 2013 state quite clearly that anyone with a leg ulcer needs to be referred to a "vascular centre" to have a colour flow venous duplex ultrasound scan and then, if found, have the underlying veins treated.

This is the subject of my book **Leg Ulcer Treatment Revolution** published in 2018 and is also the basis of some medicolegal claims that are arising from patients who have had long-term venous leg ulcers which have had an adverse effect on their lives, and who were not offered curative treatment of the underlying veins.

As far as this book is concerned, if you are prone to ulcers and already have them, or have had them before, then you will need to see a venous specialist once the lockdown or isolation is over. As before, if your lockdown rules allow you to attend medical appointments, ulcers are a medical condition that would allow you to be seen for diagnosis and treatment. If you develop an ulcer for the first time on your leg or foot during lockdown or isolation, you should seek a medical opinion immediately. The skin protects you by keeping bacteria out, and when you have a chronic open sore, it is a route for infections to get into your leg and bloodstream. In addition, ulcers can be painful (although sometimes they are remarkably pain-free) and you can lose fluid and protein from your circulation if they ooze.

The appearance of a leg ulcer or foot ulcer means that you should be referred to a specialist vascular centre or vein clinic to have a scan of your veins and possibly arteries, and then a treatment plan can be formulated. Following the NICE national guidelines in the UK, and similar guidelines elsewhere in the world, this should mean scheduling local anaesthetic treatment of the underlying veins in the very near future to start the healing process as soon as possible.

You may need some compression bandaging and dressings in the short-term whilst waiting for the treatment and during the early healing phase, but this should not be the total treatment unless you have an incurable venous disease which is really quite uncommon. The only exception to this is if you are not able to walk at all in which case compression and dressings might be your only option.

We will discuss the vein pump and the necessity for movement to make veins work after treatment later. But for now, developing a new ulcer during lockdown or isolation is one of the medical reasons related to vein health that should not wait until after the lockdown has finished before you seek help and get treatment.

Profuse bleeding of dark blood from a bulging vein on the leg or foot

One of the most serious acute complications of varicose veins or hidden varicose veins is bleeding.

When this happens, there is a sudden and often profuse bleeding of dark blood, jetting out of a vein on the lower leg or foot when standing or sitting. I have seen this happen in patients bleeding from varicose veins around ankles, foot, lower legs and in one case from a varicose vein at the knee. In almost all cases, the patient was aware that there was a varicose vein at the point where the bleed occurred.

The bleed almost always starts when the person is standing, walking or sitting. This is because in these positions, the heart is higher than the bleeding point and so there is a column of blood in the veins pressurising the blood at the point of bleeding. For this reason, when the varicose vein bursts the jet of blood is usually very impressive and quite a lot of blood can be lost quickly.

The urgent treatment for this sort of bleeding is to lie down flat and to lift the leg as high as possible. This will take all of the pressure out of the vein that is bleeding. A single finger can then be put on the bleeding point and held in place until an ambulance is called. This is certainly not something that should be left alone and, even during lockdown or isolation, is a reason to call an ambulance.

Although it is rare to die from bleeding from burst varicose veins, there have been cases reported of patients dying from this. In such cases, it is almost always the case that the patients did not seek help and, therefore, the bleeding was allowed to continue.

It is interesting to note that non-specialist doctors and nurses will often tell patients that they have "high pressure" in their varicose veins. They explain that this is what is causing the veins to bulge in the first place. Whilst this appears logical, it is not actually true.

Pressure in the veins in the majority of people only relates to where the heart is in relation to the vein. We will talk about this later in the book to help you understand veins and venous blood flow in more detail. At this point in the book, it is important to know that the higher the heart is above the vein in question, the more pressure there is in that vein. However, if the vein is higher than the heart, then there is no pressure in the vein.

This is the reason why bleeding from a varicose vein will stop if you lie down and lift the leg higher than the heart. It is also the reason why varicose veins seem to disappear when you lie down and why they look worse when you stand. It is also why people with varicose veins, hidden varicose veins or any of the other common vein problems such as venous leg ulcer all feel better when they sit down and elevate their legs.

We have now looked at most of the common symptoms and signs that occur in people with venous disease, and have given an indication as to which conditions should make you seek medical care during a lockdown or isolation and those that can be left until after the lockdown or isolation provided there is no further deterioration.

However, although venous disease is much more common in the population than often thought, there are other medical conditions that affect legs. It is not uncommon for people to blame symptoms or signs on veins that turn out to be due to other causes. I will run through the commonest of these now.

Swelling particularly of the toes on one or both sides

As we have already discussed earlier in this chapter, swelling of the legs can be due to many different causes. It is commonly associated with veins but can also be associated with lymphoedema.

The easiest distinction between swelling of the lower legs due to venous disease or lymphoedema is usually the state of the toes. In venous causes, swelling is usually maximal around the lower leg and ankle. Although it may extend onto the foot, it rarely affects the toes to any great extent.

Conversely, lymphoedema often makes the toes very swollen. In lymphoedema, toes are often so swollen that they almost appear to be moulded together in the shape of the stocking or shoe that they are within. This is the basis of the "Stemmer's sign" used by doctors and nurses to diagnose possible lymphoedema. If skin is pinched at the base of the toe, where the toe meets the foot, the skin should be thin. If it is thickened, this is a positive Stemmer's sign and indicates lymphoedema is probably present.

Lymphoedema occurs when the lymphatic channels in the leg are either blocked or not working. The lymphatic system is a little bit like the vein system because it has valves. However, the vessels are much smaller than veins, are under the skin and they also contract by themselves, "squirting" lymphatic fluid up the leg. Veins are not able to do this and have to rely on movement of the muscles and joints around them for any pumping of the venous blood.

If for any reason the lymphatics are not draining fluid up the leg, tissue fluid collects in the lower leg, foot and toes. This collection is called "oedema" and because it is due to the lymphatics not working properly, it is called lymphoedema.

In some people, there can be a combination of both venous oedema due to venous disease and also lymphoedema. Therefore, the investigation of leg swelling can be difficult.

The onset of lymphoedema with no other problem is not usually an acute medical problem that would need to be sorted out during a lockdown or isolation, but it would certainly be worth letting your family doctor know as this will need investigation later on.

Conversely, if the swelling has come on suddenly, and the leg was normal previously, then lymphoedema is unlikely and you should see a doctor urgently as in the previous sections of leg swelling above.

However, if there are any other symptoms or signs in addition to the swelling, then the advice in the previous section should be followed depending on what other symptoms or signs are present.

Swelling of both legs exactly the same on each side

We have discussed this previously, but it is worth mentioning this again in its own section. It is possible that venous disease can affect both legs identically, but it is unlikely.

Therefore, if both legs are swollen exactly the same amount, and they both started swelling at the same time, it is much less likely to be due to venous disease.

However, as in the previous section, regardless of whether it is venous or not, a sudden swelling of one or both legs, particularly if massive and associated with discomfort, should be regarded as an emergency and you should get medical assistance even during lockdown or isolation.

More minor swelling affecting just the ankles, or ankles and feet together, which is only noticeable because of the indentation by socks, and which is not associated with any other symptoms such as discomfort or pain or discolouration, is less likely to be a serious problem and can probably wait until after lockdown or isolation to be investigated, unless it worsens.

A patch of hot red skin that looks inflamed and increases in size, often causing a temperature and feeling unwell

Inflammation is the sign that the body is trying to heal.

Inflammation is characterised by redness, heat, pain and swelling (often quoted in the Latin as "rubor, calor, dolor, tumor"). Many people, including doctors and nurses, tend to think that as soon as they see inflammation there must be infection. However, some simple thinking will show why this is wrong.

For instance, if you walk into a plate glass window and bang your nose, or fall over and bang your knee, or spill hot water onto your skin, then in each of these cases the affected area will show inflammation. The area will go red, hot, will be tender or painful and will have some swelling. However, because you know the cause, you would not think the area was infected!

You have to use the same thought process in the leg. Sometimes, you will get some inflammation around the lower leg whenever you stand, because the blood is refluxing or falling the wrong way down varicose veins or hidden varicose veins and hitting the tissues in the ankle. This can cause red patches around the lower leg or ankle. This is due to simple trauma, although you cannot see the cause as you cannot see the blood flowing inside the veins. Treatment is never antibiotics but to find the source of the venous reflux, and to treat the varicose veins or hidden varicose veins. We will discuss this later.

In phlebitis or "superficial venous thrombosis" as discussed above, clots in the varicose veins or hidden varicose veins cause inflammation of the vein wall. This can cause red, hot, tender and swollen lumps to appear on the leg. As we discussed earlier, this is a clotting problem due to varicose veins and the inflammation is due to the clots and not any infection. Therefore, no antibiotics would be needed. Treatment is aimed at the clots and where they are lying, as we will discuss later.

However, there are occasions where there can be an infection in the leg. When the infection affects the skin, this is called "cellulitis". In most people, cellulitis appears as a patch of red, warm and tender skin with mild swelling in the area. Without treatment, a patch of cellulitis is likely to spread and typically starts spreading up the leg as well as outwards around it. As it worsens, it gets more tender, the patch gets bigger and often the patient will start to feel unwell with shivers and develop a temperature. It is essential that as soon as cellulitis is suspected, medical help is sought urgently as antibiotics may well be needed.

There is another form of cellulitis that presents differently. This happens in patients who also have lymphoedema. Because there is a disorder of the way fluid drains from the leg in lymphoedema, this also disorders the inflammatory response. Usually any infection would go up the lymph channels and through the lymph nodes, allowing the body to produce antibodies and T cells which fight infection. If the same infection starts in a patient with lymphoedema, the bacteria get into the bloodstream rather than the lymphatics first.

In this case, the order of events is different. With cellulitis of lymphoedema, the affected person often feels very unwell first. They think they have flu. They often have shivers and feel very "under the weather". Usually 12-24 hours later, the red patch of cellulitis will then appear on the leg.

This sort of cellulitis associated with lymphoedema is very important to recognise. Because people often feel that they have some form of "flu" first, the diagnosis of cellulitis is frequently delayed. In addition, whereas normal cellulitis is usually cured with a short course of antibiotics (typically five days) cellulitis of lymphoedema requires much longer courses of antibiotics. Three weeks is frequently the usual length of course. It is often the case where doctors will get very concerned when the cellulitis of lymphoedema is not getting better after only one week of antibiotics. They will usually give a second course, changing the antibiotic thinking there is resistance. By the end of the second week they are often panicking and worrying as to whether there is diabetes or some other problem.

Once the diagnosis has been made and a long course of antibiotics instituted, the cellulitis is usually treated effectively. Once a patient has had this, they should be given a course of antibiotics to keep with them at all times. If they ever start feeling the onset of the same sort of "flu" type symptoms again, they should start the antibiotics immediately to try to reduce the severity of the subsequent cellulitis.

Now that we have gone through the common symptoms and signs that you might experience if you have venous problems during a lockdown or isolation, we need to understand each one a little more. This will help you understand how to avoid them or, if you have them, what treatment you might need and with what urgency.

However, before we can go into the varicose venous conditions in turn, we need to understand how veins work normally.

Chapter 3

How veins work normally

Most people have a basic understanding of veins, but quickly get confused between arteries and veins when it comes to understanding how they work.

Therefore, to understand venous disease and how to keep your veins healthy, it is important to have a reasonably good understanding of the difference between arteries and veins.

Firstly, we have to consider the circulation. The whole point of having a circulation is to take oxygen and nutrients (food) to feed the tissues and organs, and then bring back the waste products for removal from the body. These waste products are basically carbon dioxide, water and several other substances such as urea. You will find popular articles and books will call these substances "toxins" but they are not really toxins. They are waste products. They can become toxic if they accumulate, but provided they are removed from the body, it is all part of normal metabolism.

This part of the circulation that takes blood to the tissues and organs and then brings the blood back again, is called the "systemic circulation".

You will not be surprised to know that in the systemic circulation, the starting point is the heart. It is actually the left side of the heart which is the stronger side. Blood full of oxygen and nutrients is pumped from the heart and into the arteries. Therefore, this is called arterial blood. Because it is full of oxygen it is bright red. Because it is pumped by the heart, it is under high pressure.

This high-pressure blood is pumped through all of the arteries to the head, arms, body, pelvis and legs. The pressure in the blood supply by the heart forces the blood through the branching arteries down to very small vessels called arterioles. From there, it flows into the capillaries in the tissues and organs.

Capillaries are very tiny blood vessels with very thin walls. These allow the oxygen and nutrients to defuse out of the arterial blood and go into the local tissue fluid. The first half of the capillary is under quite high pressure, encouraging the oxygen and nutrients to leave the blood. Therefore, from the first part of the capillary, oxygen and nutrients leave the capillary, go into the tissue fluid and then enter into the cells in the areas that need nutrition.

The cells then use the oxygen and nutrients to stay alive and to perform whatever functions they need to. For muscle cells this is movement, for gland cells it is to produce hormones or excretions, for nerve cells it is to conduct impulses and so on. The process of using oxygen and nutrients to produce energy that is then used in whatever functions the cells perform, leaving waste products such as carbon dioxide, water and other waste products like urea, is called "metabolism". Medically it is often also called "respiration" although this always causes confusion as people think respiration is breathing. Therefore, we will stick to using the term "metabolism" in this book.

The carbon dioxide, water, urea and other waste products build up in the cell. As levels of these waste products rise, they diffuse out of the cells and into the surrounding tissue fluid. As the concentration of the waste products rise in the tissue fluid, they enter the second half of the capillary which is at a much lower pressure. The waste products diffuse into the end of the capillary, just as the capillary starts joining with other capillaries to become a very small vein. This very small vein is called a "venule".

As you can see, the capillary is a very important vessel, even though it is very small. It is the part of the systemic circulation that allows the transport of oxygen and nutrients to get to the tissues and organs, and carbon dioxide, water and other waste products to be removed. The fact that it is very small is irrelevant because there are millions and millions of them throughout the whole of the body. Therefore, although each one might be small, the total surface area of all of the capillaries is huge.

Also, each capillary has an "arterial end", where the high-pressure arterial blood goes into the capillary helping force the oxygen and nutrients out into the tissues. Pressure drops off along the capillary and the other end is called the "venous end" as the capillary drains into venules and then veins. This is at much lower pressure allowing carbon dioxide, water and the waste products to defuse easily into the venous blood.

The venules all collect into small veins which then all collect into larger veins and eventually into the major venous system. Hence all of the venous blood, containing the waste products of metabolism, enters into the venous system ready to be transported back to the heart.

However, this is where we start to see the problems with understanding the venous system. Most of the arterial pressure generated by the left side of the heart has already been used to push the blood through the capillaries. By the time the blood has got to the venous end of the capillaries, there is only very little pressure left in the blood. This means, there is very little force driving the venous blood back to the heart.

When you are lying flat, there is enough pressure in the venous blood to push it back to the heart. However, as soon as you sit up or stand up, venous blood in the legs, and particularly the ankles and feet, does not have enough pressure left to push it back to the heart against gravity. This is the basis of understanding most venous problems, and so we are going to come back to this shortly.

However, before we start thinking about how blood gets back to the heart from the feet, ankles and legs, we need to complete our understanding of the circulation.

At the moment we have discussed blood leaving the left side of the heart under high pressure, full of oxygen and nutrients, being delivered to tissues and organs, and then coming back to the heart full of waste products. Clearly this cannot be the whole story, otherwise we would need an endless supply of oxygenated blood full of nutrients and there would be a build up of waste products from the venous blood, such as carbon dioxide and water.

So, what happens is that the body has a second part of the circulation system that basically "cleans" and "restocks" the blood.

All of the veins in the body keep joining together until eventually they all form one big vein called the "vena cava". This name comes from the Latin where "vena" means vein and "cava" means hollow.

The vena cava is the largest vein in the body. It drains all of the venous blood from all areas of head, arms, chest, abdomen, pelvis and legs back into the right side of the heart. The right side of the heart has a thinner muscle wall than the left side. It still pumps this blood but under less pressure than the left side of the heart.

The function of the right side of the heart is to pump blood to the lungs, where it will get rid of the carbon dioxide and pick up new oxygen. This is a second section of the circulation and, because it goes through the lungs, it is called the "pulmonary circulation".

Blood is pumped out of the right side of the heart into the pulmonary artery. This takes blood to both right and left lungs, and once again the pulmonary artery branches off into many thousands of tiny arterioles. These in turn branch into many capillaries.

Unlike the capillaries that take nutrition to the tissues and organs of the body in the systemic circulation, the capillaries in the pulmonary circulation line the little air sacs in the lung called the "alveoli". When you breathe, you take air down into the lungs and this brings oxygen into the alveoli. The wall of the alveoli is only one cell thick, the thinnest living membrane you can get. Next to it is the capillary which again is only one cell thick. Therefore, it is easy for new oxygen to diffuse through the alveoli wall and into the blood in the capillaries. It is also easy for carbon dioxide to diffuse out of the blood in the capillaries and into the alveoli space.

The continued breathing gets rid of the waste carbon dioxide and replaces the oxygen that diffuses into the blood. Blood leaving the capillaries in the pulmonary circulation is now full of oxygen and has no carbon dioxide left in it. Therefore, the blood is now ready to be sent back around the systemic circulation.

All of the little capillaries in the lung join together into venules, then into veins and eventually into the pulmonary veins. There are four of these, two on the right and two on the left. They enter directly into the left side of the heart so that the journey around the systemic circulation and then pulmonary circulation can start all over again.

Of course, this is a very simplified view of the circulation but it serves to help understand that to go around the circulation once, blood has to be pumped through the systemic circulation first, and then the pulmonary circulation afterwards.

The way that other waste products such as excess water, urea and other products of metabolism are excreted in the kidney and liver is a little more complex, but it is beyond the scope of this book to go into this in detail. This does not actually change what we need to know about the circulation.

Finally for this part of the book, we can see that we do not have to worry about flow in the arteries as these are under high pressure from a beating heart. As far as the veins are concerned, we also don't have to worry about the veins in the pulmonary circulation as these are quite short, are in the chest and next to the heart already. Therefore, the flow through them is easy and is all generated from the pressure from the right side of the heart.

The problem that we have as humans is how venous blood gets back to the heart in the systemic circulation.

We can split the body into two main areas: above the heart and below the heart. All the areas above the heart drain back into the heart by gravity when we are sitting or standing. As such we do not have to worry about blood flow in the veins of the head, neck, arms and upper chest. The majority of venous surgery, or phlebology (the study of veins) is based on how blood gets back to the heart from the feet, legs, pelvis and abdomen.

We will look at this next.

Venous return from the legs and lower body

As we saw before, the venous side of the circulation in the feet, legs and body arise from the venous end of the capillaries. Almost all of the pressure or driving force pushing the blood forwards has now been used to get the blood to the capillaries and through them. As such, there is very little pressure left to push blood from the venules back to the right side of the heart.

If you are lying down, then the pressure in the venules is sufficient to push the blood back to the heart. This is because the pressure in the entrance to the right side of the heart is almost zero, and so even the small amount of pressure in the venules is enough to push the blood through the network of veins towards the heart. Generally, veins are big and floppy, and so there is very little resistance to flow. This lets blood flow easily through the veins if there are no extra pressure problems involved.

So, when we are lying down, life is easy for venous return!

Of course, it is worth pointing out already that this is not a good strategy for the whole of a lockdown or isolation! Although flow through the veins is easy when you are lying down, it is also the slowest that venous blood flows. As you will know, not all venous problems are to do with flow. There are also venous diseases to do with blood clotting.

Lying down for extended periods of time, keeps the blood flow minimal and increases the risks of blood clots or thromboses. We are going to come back to this later in the book when we talk about deep-vein thrombosis (DVT) and "phlebitis" which we have seen is due to superficial vein thrombosis, a clot in a superficial vein.

Therefore, although lying flat helps the venous circulation when we go to bed, or if we are watching television, our venous circulation is not healthy if we don't go through episodes of standing up and walking around.

As soon as we stand up or sit up, we introduce gravity into the system.

As soon as the heart is raised above the feet, the very small pressure in the venules now has to push blood uphill, against gravity. When standing, there is just enough pressure in the venous blood to push it from the capillaries in the feet to an area just above the ankle bones. This is about 15 cm above the ground. There is not enough pressure in the venous blood to get the blood from this point up the veins in the legs, pelvis and abdomen and back to the heart.

Therefore, if there were no other forces at work, as soon as you stand or sit, your veins in your ankles and feet would start swelling until they were completely tense, and then the ankles and feet themselves would start to swell. You would then faint quite quickly as venous blood would stay in your lower legs and not get back to your heart. This would prevent any blood being pumped around the body or more importantly, to the brain. If blood does not go to the brain, you faint.

Of course, fainting is nature's way of getting blood flow back to your brain. If you faint, you fall flat, getting rid of the gravitational problem and allowing blood to flow back to your heart. From there it will be pumped onwards to supply the brain. However, a continual cycle of standing up, fainting, standing up, fainting and so on throughout the day would not be very helpful. Hence nature has developed a way to get venous blood back to the heart when you are standing or sitting, to enable you to keep living, even although there is not enough pressure in the venous blood to get back to the heart in these positions.

As we have already discussed, on the arterial side of the circulation, blood flows forward at high speed and high pressure thanks to the contraction of the heart. We have already seen that we can ignore the veins in the pulmonary circulation as they are very short, in the chest and there are no pressure problems getting the blood back to the heart. What we need, is a way of pumping blood back from the feet and legs into the right side of the heart.

We do not have a heart in our feet that continually pumps blood back from the feet or lower legs, and so we can only use the structures that are there to do the pumping. Basically, the pumping of venous blood back from the legs to the right side of the heart is performed by a combination of muscles, bones and ligaments in the feet and legs, that can compress and pressurise the veins.

A lot of simple books and articles on veins talk about the "muscle pump" in the legs, pumping the blood back through the veins to the heart. Although this is generally correct, it is worth thinking about for a couple of reasons. Apart from the heart which is a self-contained "sack" of muscle, virtually every other muscle in the body is connected to at least two other structures. This is quite obvious as the role of muscles is to create movement. A muscle sitting by itself that is not connected to anything will have no function unless it is highly specialised such as the heart muscle.

In the legs, all of the muscles connect to different bones, across joints. As most people know, there are different joints in the leg and foot. The hip joint is a ball-and-socket joint, the knee and ankle joints are basically hinge joints, and then in the foot there are a great number of joints to allow the foot to move.

In the first instance, if we think about the most basic muscle pump, we think about the calf. There are two main muscles in the calf. These attach to the top of the bones of the lower leg (tibia and fibula), run down the back of the leg into the Achilles tendon, which then inserts into the heel bone. When the calf muscle contracts, the heel is pulled up towards the back of the lower leg with a lot of force, and because of the hinge joint at the ankle this means that the front of the foot and toes is extended downwards away from the body.

We use this action when we stand on tip toes, or when we are walking. Naturally, there is an opposite set of muscles at the front of the shin that pulls the foot back upwards again. In the body, every set of muscles that makes an action has to have an opposing set of muscles to bring the action back again.

The reason that the calf muscle is so much more impressive than the muscle at the front of the lower leg is that the action of the calf muscle is against gravity. When you are standing, to stand on tiptoe's needs a lot of force, as you have to lift the whole body against gravity. Hence the calf muscle is very strong. The reverse of this is to go from tiptoe back to standing flat footed again. This is merely letting gravity work on the body, and so the muscles to do this are much less well developed.

There is a similar action of the muscles of the thigh working across the knee, and of the buttock muscles working across the hip. All of these muscles work on the bones of the legs, across the joints, to allow us to move the legs as we do.

Within the muscles of the calf and thigh, lie the deep veins of the legs. This idea of the deep veins holding the venous blood, and the muscles surrounding them, is often called the "peripheral heart". In other words, this is the main pumping force pushing blood back to the right side of the heart.

When the calf muscles or thigh muscles contract, the muscle "bulks up" which pushes on the deep veins in the legs. This forces blood upwards through the deep veins and into the veins of the pelvis and abdomen.

It is interesting to note at this point that there is also another important pump that is not quite as easy to conceive. This is the foot pump.

The foot does not have lots of bulky muscle like the calf or thigh. However, it is an arch of bones that is held in an arch by ligaments. There is one arch from the front to back, i.e. from the heel to the balls of the foot. There is also a second arch from side to side. Inside this arch are a whole lot of small veins that fill with venous blood. When you stand up, the weight of the body is transferred onto the foot, and this arch flattens. It is estimated that in a normal person, your shoe size increases by two when you stand up. This flattening of the arch squashes the veins and pumps the blood into the calf muscle pump.

Therefore, although this is not the same mechanism as the muscle pump in the calf and thigh, it is clearly part of the muscle pump of the lower limb. Not only does it feed venous blood from the foot into the calf, but it can only be activated thanks to the other muscles and bones in the legs, pelvis and trunk that enable us to stand and walk!

If you have followed this so far, you will also see that people who have flat feet will have impaired foot pumps. It is not surprising that people with flat feet are more prone to venous disease than those with normal arches. This is also the same with people who have other problems that stop normal movement of the legs.

We can now see how blood is pumped out of the lower leg and into the pelvic and abdominal veins, back towards the heart, by movement. Indeed, walking is the best movement as it coordinates the foot pump, then calf pump and then thigh pump, making sure the blood is pushed up the veins in an ordered sequence from foot to pelvis.

However, this pumping of the venous blood is only half the story. A pump is no good at all if fluid is pumped during a contraction, only to fall back to where it was before once the contraction has finished.

Therefore, a pump has two elements.

The first is the force pushing the fluid in the direction it needs to go. The second is a mechanism to keep it there, waiting for the next pump to push it further.

In the case of veins, we have already seen that the pump is the foot arch (foot pump) and the calf and thigh muscles (muscle pump). Contraction of these pumps forces blood up the deep veins of the leg and into the pelvis and abdomen. When these pumps relax, we don't want blood to fall back down the legs by gravity, undoing all of the work that the pump has just done.

This is where valves in the veins come in.

Many people know that veins have "valves" without truly understanding what they are.

Many patients who come to see me talk about "the valve" in their leg that isn't working. So, the first thing to say is that there are lots of valves in all of the veins in the legs. In the deep veins in the muscles, and also in the more superficial veins in the subcutaneous fat outside of the muscles, valves occur approximately every 8-10 cm along the veins.

As you would expect from this description, valves only let blood flow one way. In most of the veins in the foot and legs, this means that the blood is allowed to flow upwards when the pumps in the legs and foot are activated, but then close, stopping blood falling back down the leg veins by gravity when the pumps relax. However, there are other valves in the leg veins that direct the blood flow in a "one-way system" to optimise flow back to the heart. We will explore these later when we consider perforator veins.

The valves themselves are really quite delicate structures. Each valve is a pair of "leaflets" attached to the vein wall. These leaflets are arranged so that there is a free edge at the top, and they are attached to the vein wall at the sides and bottom forming a sort of "pocket". The easiest way to think of these, is to think of a pocket in a duffel coat. If you think that the coat itself is the vein wall, and the simple pocket sewn onto the outside is the valve leaflet, it gives you a fairly good idea of a vein valve.

At each venous valve, there are two of these valve "pockets" opposite each other. The valve leaflets do not actually do any work themselves, and therefore have no muscle or nerves. The free edge of the valve leaflet is pushed by different blood flows. Hence when blood is being pumped up the vein, blood rushes up past the valve leaflets, pushing them against the vein wall, and not getting in the way. Hence during active pumping, the valves have no major role.

However, when the muscle pump relaxes, and blood starts to fall back down the leg veins by gravity, the flowing blood catches the upper edge of the leaflet, with blood flowing into the "pocket" formed by the valve leaflet and the vein wall, stopping the blood flowing down the vein. The body is arranged so that the two leaflets meet in the middle of the vein, and any blood trying to fall back down the vein by gravity ends up in one valve pocket or the other. The valve is closed, and no blood can get past it.

As we saw previously, there is approximately one valve every 8-10 cm of vein in the legs, and so when standing or sitting, venous blood does not fall down the vein causing a sudden surge that would create a pressure wave impacting at the ankles.

As soon as there is any movement of foot or legs, the process begins again.

Valves working together to make a one-way system

Understanding the function of a single valve stopping blood falling down the leg due to gravity is the basic understanding of how valves work.

As with everything in medicine, it can get more complex the more you study it. One valve in one vein is easy to think about, but a network of veins with various valves is much more complex - and harder to understand when it goes wrong. However, as far as this book is concerned, we only have to think about this basic function of the vein valves, and one other.

The other slightly more complex function of the vein valves is the function of directing venous blood flow into the deep system from the superficial tissues.

Most doctors and nurses are trained to think that there are two systems of veins in the legs, the deep and superficial systems. The deep veins sit inside the muscle and account for about 90% of the blood being pumped back to the heart. The superficial veins drain venous blood from capillaries feeding the skin and subcutaneous fat, and this accounts for about 10% of the venous blood returning from the leg. However, the superficial system is split into two different systems. It is the lack of understanding of these two different systems that often leads to such bad treatments for varicose veins and leg ulcers that we see from many doctors and nurses.

The two superficial vein systems are separated into a deeper series of long straight veins that are often called venous "trunks". Many people will know these as the "saphenous" veins. They are the veins that are often used for bypass grafts as they are quite thick-walled and being long and straight, are ideal to use as grafts. They lie in their own envelope of tissue called "fascia". They are outside the muscle and therefore they are part of the superficial veins, but this fascia separates them from the subcutaneous fat and the more superficial veins. The second and more superficial part of the superficial venous system are the veins that lie under the skin and in the superficial fat, but outside of the saphenous facia.

It is most useful to think about these three systems of veins by using:

- N1 (network 1) = deep veins inside the muscle

- N2 (network 2) = truncal saphenous veins inside facia and under the subcutaneous fat

- N3 (network 3) = superficial veins outside of the saphenous facia and under the skin.

However, almost all of the venous blood leaving the leg ends up leaving through one main vein called the "femoral vein" that is in the groin. The femoral vein is part of the deep system (N1). This means that all of the venous blood in the superficial systems, both the truncal saphenous veins (N2) and superficial veins (N3) have to not only be pumped up the veins towards the heart, but also from superficial, through the muscle and into the deep N1 veins.

Most doctors and nurses have traditionally been taught that this happens because the N3 superficial veins drain into the N2 truncal veins, and these N2 veins then drain into the N1 deep veins at two main junctions. Traditionally doctors and nurses have been taught that there are 2 main N2 truncal veins, the great saphenous vein and the small saphenous vein (you will often hear doctors call these "long saphenous vein" and "short saphenous vein". However, these names changed in Europe in 2001 and in the USA in 2004 and so if you hear anyone using these old terms, they are well over a decade out of date!).

The great saphenous vein runs from the inner ankle, up the inside of the lower leg, the inside of the knee, the inside of the thigh and then dives deep through the muscle to join the N1 deep-vein in the groin at the "saphenofemoral junction" (SFJ). The small saphenous vein runs up the back of the calf and dives through the muscle behind the knees to join the deep vein (N1) at the "saphenopopliteal junction" (SPJ). Most doctors and nurses are taught that these are the two points where superficial venous blood flows into the deep veins, in order for it to be pumped up back to the heart.

However, in each leg, there are approximately 150 other veins that take blood from the superficial systems (either N2 or N3 veins), through the muscle and directly into the deep veins (N1). As these communicating veins "perforate" the tissue surrounding the muscle and the muscle itself, they are called "perforator veins", or "perforators".

Doctors and nurses like to ignore these because it is much easier to remember two big junctions that are always more or less in the same place, and much harder to look for lots of little perforating veins that can be scattered in lots of different positions all over the legs.

Now, at this point, you might not think that it is important for you to know about perforators as long as venous blood gets back to your heart. However, the understanding of the different networks of veins, and the presence of both major junctions and perforators, becomes very relevant when we talk about what goes wrong with veins, and also when we start considering whether you need treatments for certain conditions and what treatments are needed. Therefore, it is worth bringing these to your attention now.

Having looked at the basic anatomy and function of the normal leg veins, we can now start looking at the common things that go wrong with the veins and venous function.

Chapter 4

What can go wrong with veins?

At the most basic level, there are two main things that can go wrong with veins.

The first and the one that people worry about most, is that blood can clot in a vein. When blood clots inside a vein, it is called "thrombosis".

The second is that blood flow can be abnormal. The commonest cause of this in leg veins is when the valves do not work properly, a problem we have already touched upon called "venous reflux".

However, apart from venous reflux, there are two other problems that are associated with altered flow of venous blood. These are obstruction, where blood cannot flow through a narrow or blocked vein, or stasis where blood does not move sufficiently.

Of course there can be other problems such as bleeding if a varicose vein ruptures, or a leg ulcer from skin damage if venous reflux is not fixed in the long term, but these clinical problems are secondary to one or both of the basic problems listed above.

We will now go through each of these in turn.

Clots in veins - thromboses

In normal conditions, in normal people who do not have any medical problems, blood flows through the veins as a liquid. Of course, it is quite a thick liquid as it also contains cells and proteins. As everybody finds out as a child, when blood comes out of a vein such as when you fall over and graze your knee, it clots on the surface forming a scab.

This is a very important function of blood. The ability to flow through the arteries and veins as a liquid to supply oxygen, nutrients and remove waste products is essential to keep us alive, but it is also a self-healing system. When a hole is made in the system, and blood can leak out, it automatically clots and blocks up the hole.

This mechanism keeps blood in the circulation and helps keep us alive. Although everybody knows about this, many people do not then think about the next stage along. Once the blood clot has been formed to block the hole and stop leaking, the tissue has to repair. Therefore, the cells and proteins in the blood clot stimulate surrounding tissue to grow into the clot, repairing the vein wall and surrounding tissues, a process that we call "healing".

Once the healing is well under way, the clot is not needed any more. Clot on the outside of the body is a scab, and this falls off. Clot on the inside of the vein (thrombus) is removed by the body. This process is a breaking down of the clot which is medically called "thrombolysis" which literally means clot breaking down ("thrombo" = clot and "lysis" = breaking down).

So, what is it that stops the blood from clotting inside the veins normally?

Clearly the blood wants to clot when it has to, but we do not want clots to form inside arteries and veins during normal functioning. There are several reasons that blood does not clot inside the veins in normal life, but we will look at 2 of the main ones.

The first is that in normal life, blood flows fairly regularly through the arteries and veins. As we have previously seen, in the arteries this is not a problem because the heart is pumping the arterial blood at high pressure and hence high speed through the arteries. In the veins, flow is very much more variable. Provided we use the muscle pump regularly, then blood flow through the veins is also pretty good.

You may be tempted to think that as the same amount of blood flows out of the heart through the arteries to the tissue as comes back from the tissue through the veins to the heart, the flow would be the same in both arteries and veins. Unfortunately, this is not the case.

There are many more veins than arteries, and veins have a very much bigger diameter. Therefore, just in the same way that water in a river will speed up in areas where the banks get narrow, and slow down when the river gets wider, we see the same happening in the circulation. Despite the same total volume of blood flowing through the arteries and veins, the flow in the veins is very much slower. This is why we depend on exercise so much for good venous health.

Secondly, the inside of veins and arteries are lined with very special cells called "endothelial cells". These endothelial cells line the insides of all blood vessels and lie in a sheet. These sheets of cells are only one cell thick. The cells are also very flat and so are often thought to be like an internal "pavement" or "sidewalk". Not only do they form a very smooth lining, they also secrete certain chemicals that stop the blood from binding to them to start the clotting process. You can really think of the endothelial cell lining of blood vessels as a "non-stick surface for blood".

However, anything that disturbs the normal composition of the blood, flow of blood or blood vessel can lead to a situation that allows the blood to clot inside the blood vessel. As we saw before, the process of this clotting is called a "thrombosis" and the clot itself a "thrombus", although people often just call it a "blood clot".

In 1924, a scientist called Virchow described the three things that can change and cause blood to clot within a blood vessel. These are now called "Virchow's triad". Although there are three different factors, any one by itself is sufficient to start increasing the risk of thrombosis. Virchow's triad consists of:

- changes in the blood composition
- changes in the blood flow
- changes in the blood vessel wall

Any one of these things can cause thrombosis. More than one of them, increases the risk further.

Examples of each:

Changes in the blood composition - when we talk about changes in the blood composition, we mean changes in the blood constituents and perhaps viscosity. For instance, if you are on holiday in a very hot country, you will become dehydrated if you do not keep up with your fluid input. Hence your blood will become more concentrated and more viscous. This can be worsened if you drink alcohol on holiday because alcohol is a diuretic. This means it is a drug that makes you pass more urine than the fluid you drink. Therefore, even though you are drinking fluid, you are actually getting more dehydrated. If you have an illness and a high temperature, you can both get an increase in viscosity from dehydration and also increased proteins and cells as your body starts producing antibodies and white blood cells.

Other things that change the blood composition include cigarette smoke which increases the protein called fibrinogen making the blood more viscous and therefore "sticky", certain drugs and in particular the oral contraceptive pill with high oestrogen levels, and some cancers. We are not sure why some cancers make the blood stickier, but we do know this happens.

Lastly, some people are just born with different proteins in their blood which increase the risk of clotting. This is called a "thrombophilia" which simply means "clot liking" ("thrombo" = clot, "philia" = "liking" or "loving"). Many of these are inherited and you might often hear of certain thrombophilia's such as Factor V Leiden (pronounced Factor five Leiden), protein S deficiency or protein C deficiency which are some of the more commonly inherited thrombophilias.

Changes in the blood flow - changes in blood flow that are more likely to cause clots particularly in the veins, are a slowing down of the flow, reversal of flow or turbulence.

As we have discussed before, and as is fairly obvious, the more you exercise, the faster the blood flow in the veins. The more you sit or lie still and don't move, the slower the blood flow, particularly if the legs are hanging down and gravity cannot get the blood back out of the ankles.

Turbulence in veins can happen for different reasons. The commonest cause of turbulence in veins is having varicose veins. We will discuss this later in this chapter when we talk about blood flow. However, at this point it is worth noting that when you have varicose veins, or even hidden varicose veins, turbulence happens for different reasons.

Firstly, the blood flow reverses from upwards to refluxing downwards. The second is that there may be turbulence during reflux as the failed valves might partially close. Refluxing blood flow, squeezing past this partial obstruction will be turbulent. Thirdly, the vein wall is dilated in different areas, causing the blood to tumble into cavities and then back to narrow sections of the vein. This causes turbulence and increases the risk of clots.

Other causes of turbulence occur when there is something interrupting the smooth flow of blood in the vein. This might be something inside the vein itself such as a thrombus that is already there, causing more thrombus to form, or it might be a medical device such as a "drip" - medically called a "cannula" in an arm vein.

In the veins in the pelvis, there can be structures inside the lumen of the vein, causing an obstruction to the flow. This can occur if there has been a previous deep vein thrombosis, and scar tissue has been left behind that can cause a partial membrane across the inside of the vein, getting in the way of the normal flow. Another recognised problem is called a "non-thrombotic iliac vein lesion" (or NVIL) which can occur in the large veins in the pelvis. This is often thought to be a partially formed valve that is not used in humans anymore but can leave a "web" that partially obstructs the vein.

Another cause of obstruction to smooth flow can be from something pushing on the vein from the outside. There are several areas of the body where the veins can get trapped under different structures. In the pelvis, on the left side, the artery to the right leg passes from the aorta and over the front of the left vein in the pelvis (called the common iliac vein) as it travels towards the right groin. Although in most people this does not cause a problem, in some people, the artery can push back on the vein and crush it against the spine. When this occurs, it is called the "May Thurner syndrome". This has been an area that is gaining a lot of interest amongst venous surgeons and phlebologists.

Changes in the blood vessel wall - as we discussed previously, veins and arteries have a specialist lining called the "endothelium" or layer of "endothelial cells". This single layer of cells lines the inside of the vessels and has some very special properties. The first, is that it secretes substances to stop the blood clotting on it in normal circumstances as previously noted. A second special property is that it has a layer of molecules on the surface called the "Glycocaylix". This is a layer of molecules that sits on the endothelial cells, helping them function properly.

Blood flowing over the endothelial cells and the glycocaylix causes a "shear stress" between the blood flow and the wall itself. The faster the flow, the greater the shear stress.

Shear stress is actually very healthy for the blood vessel wall, both in arteries and veins, as this shear stress causes the endothelial cells to produce a substance called nitric oxide. This goes into the wall, keeping the artery and vein wall healthy and soft, reducing problems such as inflammation and "hardening of the arteries". Reduced flow reduces the amount of shear stress and also reduces the level of this healthy nitric oxide.

Also, it appears that substances that get into the blood from cigarette smoke seem to destroy the nitric oxide. This is one of the reasons why cigarette smoking is so disastrous for the cardiovascular system and circulation.

Of course, as far as veins are concerned, the commonest cause of having vein walls that are damaged is having varicose veins. In varicose veins, the vein wall is stretched by the blood flowing the wrong way, damaging it and causing the dilations which we call "varicose veins". When the vein wall is stretched and dilated, it is not healthy anymore and so is more likely to allow a clot to form on it. In addition, people who have had varicose veins for a long time or have had previous clots such as phlebitis or deep vein thrombosis, will often have residual scars in the vein wall. The scars stop the vein wall from dilating normally, and give an abnormal surface making future clots more likely to form in the same place.

Blood clots in leg veins - phlebitis, superficial venous thrombosis and deep vein thrombosis

Many people are understandably worried when a doctor tells them that they have a "clot" in their leg veins.

As we have seen, if the blood clot forms inside a blood vessel, medically we call it a thrombosis, and the clot, a thrombus. Although thromboses can form in the arterial system, they are much rarer than thromboses in the venous system, and not so relevant for this book. As such we are going to concentrate on venous thromboses.

Until 2012, most doctors and nurses thought that it was quite easy to differentiate between the two main different sorts of venous thrombosis in leg veins.

If the thrombus was in a deep vein, it was a "deep vein thrombosis" or a "DVT" and was serious.

If the thrombosis was in a superficial vein, it was called "phlebitis" (or more accurately "superficial venous thrombophlebitis") although now most of us venous experts prefer to call this a "superficial venous thrombosis". For generations this was thought to be completely benign.

However, our understanding of leg veins and venous thromboses in leg veins has changed considerably. As previously alluded to, despite guidelines published in the USA and UK in 2012, most doctors and nurses seem to be unaware of these changes.

Therefore, we will look through these two different conditions now.

1 - Deep vein thrombosis (DVT)

As we discussed in Chapter 3, the deep veins (N1 veins) lie inside the muscles of the legs. They take about 90% of the venous blood back from the legs to the right side of the heart. This then flows through the pulmonary circulation to the lungs.

If for any of the reasons we discussed above, a clot forms in these deep veins, it is called a deep vein thrombosis. Because thrombosis in a vein causes inflammation, there will usually be some discomfort.

In Chapter 2 we briefly considered how the size and position of a deep vein thrombosis might vary the symptoms and signs that a person might feel or see. We will look at this in a bit more detail now.

The level of discomfort will depend on the size of the clot and where it is. In addition, a deep vein thrombosis might completely block a vein (occlusive) or might only partially block it (non-occlusive). Obviously blocking a vein will cause swelling below the area of the blockage. This swelling might cause some tightness and discomfort in addition to any obvious swelling that might be seen externally. Irritation of the vein in the muscle can also cause pain on contraction of the muscle.

Therefore, we can see that clots in the lower leg veins are likely to cause a tender swollen calf and lower leg. Clots in the thigh are likely to cause discomfort of the whole of the leg from the thigh downwards, and more considerable swelling. Clots in the iliac veins in the pelvis, can cause massive leg swelling as well as considerable pain and discomfort.

In addition to the local problems caused by the thrombosis irritating the vein and local muscle, and the obstruction causing the swelling below that level, there is also a risk that parts of the thrombus can break off, travelling through the venous system into the right side of the heart and lung. This is commonly called "a clot to the lung" or medically a "pulmonary embolism" ("pulmonary" = lungs, "embolism" = "abnormal object within the normal blood flow").

As such, people have become paranoid about "DVT". However, there are some things that are worth knowing. As you might expect, the deep veins are a tapering system. This is because all of the way along the veins, more veins are joining in and bringing waste blood from surrounding tissues. Therefore, there is increasing amounts of venous blood to return to the heart the higher up the leg we go.

In the calf, there are six deep veins, all of them only a couple of millimetres in diameter. They all join together about the knee into a vein called the popliteal vein which is larger, being about 5 mm in diameter. The vein in the thigh is called the femoral vein, and again is slightly larger than the popliteal vein. In the groin, the vein leaving the leg is called the common femoral vein and is really quite large at this stage. The iliac veins inside the pelvis are even bigger.

Therefore, not only is the amount of pain and distribution of swelling dependent on which vein has thrombosed, but also the volume of the thrombus itself is drastically different depending where it occurs. A thrombus in the calf vein has a very small volume, and even if the whole thing were to break off and fly to the lungs, it is unlikely that anyone would notice it. On the other hand, a clot in the pelvic veins (iliac veins) is going to be very large because the vein is over a centimetre in diameter, and if this were to break off and embolise up the veins through the right side of the heart and into the lungs it is likely to cause a very significant pulmonary embolism and could even cause death.

Therefore, not all deep vein thromboses are the same. This is why treatment of a deep vein thrombosis will change depending on where the deep vein thrombosis is in the legs. It is also why it is essential to have a high-quality colour flow duplex ultrasound scan to know exactly the position and extent of the deep vein thrombosis as soon as possible, in order to get the optimal treatment.

One other thing that it is probably worth knowing is that thromboses can grow. For instance, if you develop a clot on the vein wall at a certain point in the leg, for any reason in particular, blood flow in the local area will be disturbed. Immediately the thrombosis occurs, blood flow in the vein around it starts changing.

If the thrombus does not completely block the vein (called a "non-occlusive" thrombus), then the blood flow in the same vein will have to speed up locally to get past the thrombus. Once the blood has passed the clot, it will slow down and become turbulent. Hence the vein wall will have changed because of the presence of thrombus, and the flow would have changed both speeding up at the point of the clot and then slowing down and being turbulent after the thrombus. These changes cause more blood to clot on the part of the thrombus downstream of the flow, meaning that the clot starts to grow in length. This is called "extension of the thrombus".

This process can continue until the whole vein becomes occluded, or indeed the whole process might start off with an immediate total occlusion of the vein. Whichever way it occurs, once the vein becomes occluded, there is no flow in that section until the next major tributary bringing blood flow into the vein. Therefore, the whole segment that has no flow in it, will clot off immediately. This will cause a very large thrombus extension.

In this way, a small thrombosis in a deep vein can extend quite rapidly. In many cases, the original thrombus starts healing and can be quite hard. New thrombus, like any new blood clot, is soft and spongy. When a pulmonary embolism occurs, it is often the soft spongy "tail" or extension that flies off to the right side of the heart and the lungs, although in other cases it is the whole thrombus itself. This is why when patients turn up with a pulmonary embolism, sometimes it is impossible to find the deep vein thrombosis that caused it, while on other occasions, the deep vein thrombosis is still present in the leg or pelvic veins.

It also explains why some pulmonary emboli are worse than others. A small clot flying into a small part of the lungs may have very little effect. However, a substantial clot that is very long (sometimes 15 cm or so long and 1 cm or so diameter) that travels up to the right side of the heart, can get caught here even before it gets to the lungs. This can cause the heart to fail to pump properly. In this situation, the heart can undergo acute heart failure, and this failure to pump means that a patient can die within minutes. This is usually what happens when you hear of people "dropping dead" from a "clot to the lungs".

Although this is very scary, it is obviously the very worst-case scenario. Most people who have deep vein thromboses only have them in the calf veins or veins below the knees. Provided treatment is started to stop any more clot forming and extending the clot, these sorts of deep vein thromboses rarely cause a problem either acutely or in the long term.

However, as you can see, it is essential to know the position of the deep vein thrombosis and the size of it as soon as possible to get the right treatment. We will come back to this later.

2 - "Phlebitis", superficial venous thrombophlebitis and superficial venous thrombosis

To be able to understand "phlebitis", superficial venous thrombophlebitis and superficial venous thrombosis, we need to have a good understanding of the superficial veins of the legs.

As we saw in Chapter 3, we now recognise 3 networks of veins in the legs.

To recap, the deep veins are the N1 ("Network one") and are in the anatomical compartment one (or AC1) which means inside the muscles of the legs. The long "truncal" veins (often called the "axial" veins) that run up the leg just above the muscle and that cannot be seen from the surface, are the N2 ("Network two") lying in the saphenous fascia or anatomical compartment 2 (AC2). The multitude of veins lying under the skin and in the subcutaneous fat are the N3 ("Network three") with the subcutaneous fat being the anatomical compartment 3 (AC3).

This system of defining two different networks of superficial veins is not just being pedantic. There are real differences between these veins that both affect patients and also the way we treat vein problems. It is the lack of understanding of these two systems that still results in many patients getting very bad venous surgery.

Indeed, recently there was an argument at a UK national "vein meeting" between two doctors who were vascular (arterial) surgeons and not vein specialists, who were arguing whether compression works after sclerotherapy. Both had opposing views as to whether compression should be used or not.

If only they understood the difference between N2 veins and N3 veins, they would not have to have had the argument! N2 veins have very thick walls and do not respond well to treatment with sclerotherapy. Also, they lie deeper in the AC2 and cannot be compressed with compression stockings. Conversely, N3 veins are thin walled, respond very well to sclerotherapy and, as they lie more superficially in the AC3, can be compressed by compression stockings. If the vascular surgeons who only treat a few patients with vein problems each week listened to venous experts who specialise in treating patients with venous disease alone, they would find that a lot of the questions they still argue about have already been answered.

One of the ways that many people find helpful to visualise the difference between N2 and N3 veins is bypass surgery. Most people are aware that you can remove the long straight veins from the lower leg for heart bypass surgery, or the same vein right up the leg for bypass surgery in the leg, used in patients with blocked leg arteries. However, most people would also be surprised if doctors used the little green veins that are seen branching just under the skin for this sort of bypass. It is the N2 veins that are deep under the fat but outside of the muscle that are used for the bypasses whereas the superficial N3 veins would be useless for this sort of surgery.

So why is this important?

When blood clots in a superficial vein, it causes inflammation. As we have seen, inflammation has four components. These are:

- redness
- heat
- pain
- swelling

Whenever you suffer any trauma, infection, chemical burn or anything else that damages your body, your body responds by starting an inflammatory process.

The local blood vessels dilate, bringing more blood and nutrients to the area, making the area go red. Not only does the increased blood flow bring more nutrients, it also brings more white blood cells and antibodies. If the problem is infection, these will fight the infection. If the problem is dead tissue or dying tissue, the white cells will start to eat away the dead tissue to start the process of replacing it.

The area becomes tender because when the body starts an inflammatory process, it deliberately secretes chemicals that cause pain. This stops you from using the area while the body gets on with the important process of healing. Finally, the swelling is due to the extra tissue fluid brought about by the extra blood supply. In addition, there may be a lump caused by the tissue that is being removed as it is packed full of white blood cells which are trying to eat it away.

Let us now think about a clot occurring in an N3 vein just under the skin surface on the calf. It is likely that this vein was a varicose vein, and the clot formed because the wall was stretched and hence the flow was disturbed. The clot forms inside the vein as a thrombus. This irritates the vein wall causing acute inflammation. The vein becomes very inflamed, which spreads into the local tissues. White blood cells go into the blood clot trying to help resolve the clot and trying to fix the vein wall. Now there is an inflammatory lump in the calf. Please note this point, there is no infection at all. The whole process is because of a local blood clot forming in a superficial vein.

So, you might have noticed a varicose vein and suddenly, you find a red, hot, painful and swollen lump where the varicose vein used to be. When you touch it, it is hard. Unfortunately, because of the lack of understanding noted above, doctors, nurses and patients often reach for antibiotics. Not surprisingly, these have no effect at all. Indeed, they may make matters worse by giving the patient a fungal infection due to changing the bacteria in the gut and on the skin and may well lead to resistance.

Some people who have had "phlebitis" claim that antibiotics have worked over the course of a few days to a week. However, in these cases, either there was a misdiagnosis, or the inflammation was already working and would have worked whether the antibiotics were given or not. Basically, antibiotics have no place in the treatment of superficial venous thrombosis.

It might be useful to understand why the term "phlebitis" is used. When a superficial venous thrombosis occurs like this, the resulting inflammation in the vein is naturally called "phlebitis" (literally inflammation of the vein; "phleb" = vein, "itis" = inflammation).

Unfortunately, many people including doctors and nurses will call any inflammation in the legs "phlebitis". For instance, patients who have had venous reflux from varicose veins or hidden varicose veins for a long time, will often get inflammation in the skin on the inside of their lower leg, just above the ankle. If this redness is left for a long time, it will eventually become a brown stain. If the venous reflux is not stopped, it will eventually destroy the skin causing a venous leg ulcer. This inflammation of the skin is variously called "venous eczema", "venous skin changes" or if it goes brown, "haemosiderin". It is an inflammation of the skin and the underlying skin. It is not an inflammation of the veins and is not phlebitis at any stage of the progression.

Because of this confusion, we try not to use the word "phlebitis" and try to be more precise calling a clot in the superficial veins "superficial venous thrombophlebitis". As you can see this literally means an inflammation of the veins caused by a clot, in the superficial veins. However, because the word phlebitis has so many poor connotations, and so many doctors still think "itis" means infection rather than inflammation, to try to get doctors, nurses and patients to stop thinking about infection and antibiotics, we now call this condition "superficial venous thrombosis".

Now putting together what we have understood about N2 and

N3 veins, along with the description above of superficial venous thrombosis, you can start to see that a clot in the "superficial veins" can have many different presentations and outcomes, just the same as a deep vein thrombosis can in the deep N1 system.

To simplify things, if the thrombosis occurs in a small vein near the surface (AC3), then the patient will notice a small lump that is red, hot, tender and swollen. The vein is also likely to be hard and the lump can be felt if it is near the surface. If several connected superficial veins are affected, then there may be quite extensive hard lumps, all of them red, hot, tender and swollen.

However, if the thrombosis is affecting the N2 veins, then the signs and symptoms are quite different. Because the N2 veins are long and straight and lie deep under the skin and within their own fascia (AC2), the usual presentation is pain or discomfort. This runs up the leg on the inside in a long line (if it is in the great saphenous vein), or up the back of the calf in a line (if it is in the small saphenous vein).

Sometimes if the inflammation is very pronounced, a red line can be seen on the skin. However, the vein is so deep that in many cases no redness can be seen on the surface. For the same reasons, localised heat and localised swelling may not be found, although tenderness is almost always there particularly if the area is pushed with the fingers.

Obviously because all of the veins are connected, there can be a thrombus that extends from N3 to N2 veins, and indeed, can extend into N1 veins. If it extends into N1 veins, then parts of the thrombus can fly off, causing a pulmonary embolism. This was the revolutionary finding that was noted in 2012 – that superficial venous thrombosis can cause pulmonary embolism.

So, to bring this section to a close, there are three very major points we have to be aware of.

The first is that "phlebitis", or more correctly superficial venous thrombosis, can have varying signs and symptoms, depending on which veins are affected.

The second is that it should not be taken as a simple condition, as some patients will be at risk of extension into the deep veins (N1) and pulmonary embolism to the lungs.

Finally, antibiotics are never the treatment for superficial venous thrombosis.

We will come back to the correct investigations and treatments for this condition later in the book.

Abnormal flow in the veins - valve failure

The second major thing that can go wrong with veins is that flow can be abnormal within them. There are three major reasons that this can happen:

- reflux
- obstruction
- stasis

In the rest of this chapter, we are going to concentrate on venous reflux as this is such an important problem in venous surgery, and it affects some 30-40% of the adult population.

However, we will address obstruction and stasis very briefly first to enable us to concentrate on reflux.

As far as obstruction is concerned, we have already discussed this earlier in this chapter. Obstruction can be partial or complete and can be inside the lumen of the vein, caused by scar tissue in the wall of the vein or something pushing on the outside of the vein. However, the results are a reduction in flow and maybe a complete blockage of the flow. We will talk about treatments of obstruction later in the book.

Venous stasis means blood flowing very slowly or blood moving forwards and backwards and not moving much at all in the veins. We've already discussed that venous blood needs to flow away from the tissues, up through the veins and back through the right side of the heart to the lungs so that it can get rid of the carbon dioxide, water and other waste products of metabolism. Although venous stasis makes you think that the blood might just sit completely still in the veins, it cannot do this. If blood does not move, then it clots, and this will become a thrombus.

Venous stasis means that blood is not pumped forward up the veins in the normal way. There must be just enough movement in the blood, whether forwards or rocking forwards and backwards, to stop the blood from clotting and forming a thrombus.

The reason venous stasis causes problems is very interesting. If you think of blood only as a liquid, then blood accumulating around the ankles should not really cause much problem. It might cause some swelling as more blood accumulates, but you wouldn't naturally think it would damage the body.

However, as we have already talked about, blood is not only a liquid but contains many cells. It carries the waste products from the cells being carbon dioxide, water, and other waste products like urea. When carbon dioxide, urea or other waste products accumulate, they can reach concentrations that are poisonous to the body. In addition, the cells in the blood all have to stay alive themselves. Therefore, the red blood cells and white blood cells in the venous blood continue to metabolise any remaining oxygen and nutrients to stay alive, producing even more carbon dioxide, water and other waste products.

Carbon dioxide dissolves in water to form carbonic acid. The more carbon dioxide in the blood, the more acidic it becomes. In addition, the more carbon dioxide, the more metabolism, and therefore the more other metabolic wastes that will be in the blood. This combination of increasingly acidic blood with increasing concentrations of waste products of metabolism, starts irritating the vein wall if the blood is not removed from them. Hence, venous stasis means that this blood fails to get out of the veins, particularly around the ankles. This increases the damage to the vein walls and surrounding tissues, increasing the inflammation of the subcutaneous tissue and eventually the skin itself.

This inflammation can result in venous eczema, or the typical venous skin damage leading to leg ulcers, or can even start causing thrombosis in any of the veins around the ankle, deep or superficial.

Venous reflux

In the last chapter, we have previously talked about how blood is pumped out of the leg veins by movement, and how it is dependent upon a chain of valves in every vein of the leg to make sure venous blood only flows one way. Blood being pumped up the veins cannot fall back down the veins when the muscles relax. Blood flowing from superficial veins into deep veins cannot flow back out into the superficial veins. Hence in the normal patient we have a one-way system, driven by a combination of movement and valves.

Unfortunately, these valves can fail. When these valves fail, blood can fall the wrong way through the failed valves. This is called venous reflux, and the affected vein is said to be "incompetent".

Another term that is often used is "insufficiency". When a patient has enough valves that have failed in a leg to cause venous disease, such as varicose veins, aching, tired legs, swelling of the ankles, red or brown stains around the ankles, leg ulcers, superficial venous thrombosis or bleeding, then it is often said that the patient has "chronic venous insufficiency". This merely means that some of the veins are incompetent due to different patterns of valves having failed and not working properly.

Traditionally, doctors and nurses are only taught the simplest facts about venous disease. Because there is very little formal training in venous surgery, most doctors never find out more. This is a major reason why so many patients who have varicose vein treatments get such bad results.

As we have seen, the usual teaching for doctors and nurses is that there is only a deep system and a superficial system. The deep system rarely goes wrong. They are taught that when it does, and the valves fail in the deep system, this causes venous leg ulcers, and nothing can be done to cure this. The only treatment is said to be compression dressings. The superficial system often goes wrong. The usual teaching is that when valves fail in the superficial system, the result is varicose veins which are only cosmetic. Traditional teaching is that these can be treated, but it is only a cosmetic problem.

Furthermore, such outdated teaching indicates that if treatment for varicose veins is undertaken, it is either the great saphenous vein or the small saphenous vein that needs treatment, or both. Such teaching gives the impression that provided you know which of these veins to treat, or treat both if needed, you will get the right treatment.

Unfortunately, all of this simple understanding has been shown to be complete rubbish.

First of all, most venous leg ulcers occur because valves fail in the superficial system, not the deep system. As we have seen previously, the superficial system is actually made up of two sections, the N2 truncal veins and the N3 more superficial veins. In addition to these, there are the perforating veins. Research is now clearly shown that when there is reflux in the N2 superficial venous system and/or incompetence of perforator veins, a gradual deterioration of venous function happens in the leg.

This gradual deterioration starts off with varicose veins being visible in about half the people who are affected, with the other half having the same venous reflux but nothing visible on the surface. If nothing is done to stop the reflux, the usual trend of deterioration is:

- aching and tired legs that only improve when the legs are elevated
- swelling around the ankles
- venous eczema usually over the lower legs but occasionally over the knees or thighs
- red or brown skin stains around the inner aspect of the lower leg either just above the ankle or around the ankle
- skin breakdown and an open sore developing called a venous leg ulcer

Other complications can include bleeding from veins or thromboses in the veins.

It is now known that most venous leg ulcers can be permanently cured by venous experts treating the underlying reflux in the N2 veins and/or refluxing perforating veins. However, despite the huge improvement of quality-of-life this would lead to patients and their families, and the huge savings it would make for health services to stop having to bind so many legs, paying for dressings, compression and nursing time, most people with venous leg ulcers still only get offered compression dressings.

Moreover, even though we now know the progression of varicose veins or hidden varicose veins to all of these problems, most people only seek or get referred for help when the disease has progressed sufficiently enough to start causing skin damage, thromboses or ulceration. If patients got treated when they started getting symptoms, as the UK national guidelines suggest, then this whole progression of disease would be prevented.

However, that also depends upon the right treatment being performed.

Although patients concentrate on which technique doctors use, such as laser, radiofrequency, sclerotherapy injections, medical glue, high intensity focused ultrasound etc. none of these are any good at all if the wrong veins are being targeted.

Despite all the research that has been done in the venous world, most doctors and nurses still only check for reflux in the great saphenous vein and the small saphenous vein. Moreover, they only treat reflux in the great saphenous vein or small saphenous vein. This is one of the major reasons why you hear people say "varicose veins always come back".

However, this is not true.

If all of the problem veins are found and treated, then the results can be excellent. Indeed, our own recurrence rate is between 3 and 4.5% per year, which as we will see later, is the natural deterioration rate of people who have varicose veins in their family. It is impossible to get lower than this.

So, what patterns of superficial venous disease are there?

If the long veins in the N2 system become incompetent due to the valves failing along the length of the vein, then blood falls down the vein by gravity as soon as you sit or stand. Because this reflux is due to gravity, we call this "passive" reflux. Some venous surgeons call this "diastolic" reflux meaning that the muscles are relaxed. I personally do not like the term diastolic as I think this relates more to the heart and so I favour the term passive reflux.

So when a traditionally trained doctor or nurse thinks about varicose veins, they will be looking for passive reflux in the great saphenous vein, refluxing from the groin down the inside of the thigh to the inside of the knee and then to the ankle, or the small saphenous vein, refluxing from behind the knee, down the middle of the calf to the outside ankle.

However, we now know that passive reflux also affects veins inside the pelvis called the gonadal veins (ovarian veins in the female and testicular veins in the male) and the internal iliac veins, as well as the anterior accessory and posterior accessory saphenous veins in the upper thigh. The anterior accessory saphenous vein is the one that causes varicose veins on the front of the thigh going to the outside of the knee and is often ignored by doctors treating varicose veins as only part of their full-time job.

The second sort of reflux is called active reflux. This is explained more fully in my book "**Understanding Venous Reflux - the cause of varicose veins and venous leg ulcers**" but I will try and explain it simply here. If you consider a perforating vein at the level of the calf, it is going straight from the N3 vein just under the skin, draining blood through the subcutaneous fat, perforating through the fascia around the muscle and the muscle itself and draining into the deep vein. There is at least one valve along this vein making sure blood only goes inwards.

When the calf muscle contracts, blood is squirted straight up the deep N1 vein towards the heart. It cannot squirt back along the perforating vein towards the skin, because of the perforating vein valve.

However, if the valve in the perforating vein has failed, and the perforating vein is incompetent, when the calf muscle contracts, the blood is squirted both up the N1 vein towards the heart along with all the other blood in the deep vein, but also a significant amount is pumped back out of the perforating vein into the N3 vein just under the skin surface.

You can imagine the pressure in the deep veins in the calf during muscle contraction by considering the pressure needed to pump blood up to the heart from the calf, against gravity. This same very high pressure is squirting the blood outwards along the incompetent perforating vein, impacting the N3 vein just under the skin. Not surprisingly, this very high pressure jet of blood causes damage, which might be a dilation of the vein showing a varicose vein, or might dilate an area of skin veins causing telangiectasia (often called thread veins or spider veins) or, if left for a long time, may even end up causing inflammation in the skin resulting in venous eczema, red stains, brown stains and eventually leg ulcers.

As we have noted before, there are approximately 150 perforating veins in the leg. Any of these can become incompetent.

Therefore any colour flow duplex ultrasound scan for venous reflux disease in the leg that does not include great saphenous vein, small saphenous vein, anterior accessory and posterior accessory saphenous veins, any duplicate systems, any sign of veins coming from the pelvis into the legs, and all 150 perforating veins, including checking the deep veins are working, is inadequate. It is amazing how many patients report to us that they have been to see doctors who do their own scans, and the whole scan only took a couple of minutes! It is not surprising that these are the sorts of doctors that only treat the main two saphenous veins, ignoring all other causes of venous reflux.

I hope that this explanation has given you an understanding of how important the valves are to pump blood back to the heart, and the difference between passive and active reflux. Also, I hope I have given an understanding about the myriad of different combinations of reflux in different veins, both active and passive that may coexist causing venous disease in any particular leg.

When a patient has venous disease due to venous reflux, which is the commonest form of venous disease and affects approximately one third of the whole adult population, it is essential to work out exactly what pattern of reflux they have in each affected leg. With so many combinations possible, it really means that we now have to treat each individual patient as an individual pattern, and tailor treatments precisely to each individual patient.

This also shows how ridiculous it is to think of a "standard" varicose vein operation. The same symptoms and signs can have a multitude of underlying causes, all taking completely different lengths of times and techniques to correct.

Now that we have discussed what can go wrong with the veins, we can move on to thinking about which sorts of patients are at more risk of venous disease than others, particularly during a lockdown or isolation.

Chapter 5

Who is at risk of venous problems during a lockdown or in isolation?

Whenever we think about patients at risk for a certain condition, we always like to separate the factors into those that you cannot change, and those that you can.

As we have seen previously, although the symptoms and signs vary considerably, most of the urgent problems that can occur from venous disease arise from either blood clots (thromboses) forming in certain veins, or pre-existing venous reflux disease worsening.

Many of the risk factors that we are going to discuss will be obvious to you if you have read the previous chapters and understood how veins work and what can go wrong with them.

However, we will go through some of the major risk factors for venous disease and discuss each one briefly. It may interest you that I am not going to discuss sex, as contrary to a lot of the out-of-date research, almost all of the modern research shows there is very little difference between males and females in the incidence of venous disease.

Moreover, it will surprise you that I'm not going to start with age, as many people still think that varicose veins and venous disease is a problem of "old people". As you'll see, this is not the case.

Family history

One of the strongest indicators of whether you will get venous disease is your family history. This is particularly true for venous reflux but can also be true for thrombosis.

There has been quite a lot of research done looking at who gets "varicose veins" and there is quite a strong link to a family history of the condition. Research from a major population study has suggested that a normal person has approximately a 1.6% risk every year of developing varicose veins, where as someone who has varicose veins in their family has somewhere between a 3.0 and 4.5% risk of developing varicose veins each year.

This has led to some people to call the risk of getting varicose veins "genetic". However, that isn't quite right. If it was only genetic, you'd always get varicose veins in both legs and also in all of the veins. The fact that we often get varicose veins only on one leg, and almost always only in a certain pattern of veins, shows that you inherit a familial tendency to varicose veins but then other factors act on the body to cause varicose veins to develop in some veins but not others.

Also, just because valves fail in the leg vein, doesn't mean to say you will definitely get venous disease. For instance, if you had one valve or two valves fail in the middle of a long N2 truncal vein, or several valves fail in several different superficial N3 veins, you might well have quite a lot of venous reflux but not enough in one area to cause any clinical problem.

Conversely, if just one valve fails in a particular perforator, this can go on to cause varicose veins and, in some cases, even skin damage and worse. Therefore, although we know that varicose veins and a lot of venous disease do come from valves that fail, it is possible that some valves can fail in some people without venous disease occurring, especially in the short-term.

As we discussed previously, the chance of developing thromboses can increase if you inherit certain genetic traits related to blood coagulation such as Factor V Leiden, protein S or protein C or others - the thrombophilias. However, a great number of people who develop deep vein thrombosis or superficial vein thrombosis have no family history at all of the condition, and the clots have only developed because of local problems such as immobility, dehydration, major surgery, cancer or other things that are not necessarily directly attributable to family history.

Varicose veins are quite interesting in this respect. As we have already said, the risks of getting varicose veins increase with a strong family history. However, you can get them without having any relatives with varicose veins at all. Varicose veins can then cause thromboses due to Virchow's triad, although we would not call this resulting thrombosis a familial problem.

So generally, severe varicose veins and the complications of these such as leg ulcers can run in families. Also inherited genetic thrombophilias that cause deep vein thromboses can also run in families. A strong family history may well indicate a problem, but not having a family history does not mean you are not going to get a venous problem!

Age

Almost all deteriorating diseases worsen with age.

Children and adolescents rarely get venous thromboses. Indeed, it is usually only those that are very sick or have some major risk factor that will get a venous thrombosis at all. However, the risks of developing venous thromboses increase with age throughout life.

It is thought that everybody has an underlying risk of venous thrombosis that increases with age. Some people will be at high risk and will develop a thrombosis quite early in their life, usually at a time when there is a stress to the system such as dehydration, surgery or one of the other causative conditions we discussed earlier.

This is worked out by the fact that some people will have a certain stress early in their lives, and not develop a deep vein thrombosis, but later in their lives subject to the same stress, they will develop a deep vein thrombosis. As such, the causes of deep vein thrombosis we discussed before are not usually the only reason for deep vein thrombosis but are an additional stress on a system that already has an underlying propensity to clot.

If you are lucky and have a very low propensity to clot throughout your life due to your genetic make-up, and perhaps your activity, diet etc, then a certain stress that might cause a deep vein thrombosis in someone else may well not cause the same problem in you.

This is one of the complexities of medicine. Although we all like to know that certain things are bad for us, or that certain activities, drugs, events and so on will cause a problem, medical conditions are often much more complex. The same stress on the whole population of people will cause some people to have a complication but not others.

This is because almost all diseases are multifactorial.

When it comes to venous reflux disease and age, we know that varicose veins and hidden varicose veins worsen with age. Many studies have shown that in susceptible people, the first valves often fail at childhood or early teens. The reflux then continues to deteriorate and cause clinical symptoms over time. However, we also know that some people never have valve failure at all and have perfect veins to the ends of their long lives. As such, once again, although time and hence age will worsen any valve failure, it is very variable as to whether it will cause a clinical problem at all in any particular person, and if it does, at what age this will start to show.

In my own personal experience, I have had to operate on a 12-year-old boy with some of the most severe varicose veins I have ever seen. Not surprisingly, he had a very strong history of varicose veins with his mother and father both coming to seek opinions from me having had many varicose vein operations performed elsewhere in the past.

Hence although we can generally say that venous disease, both thromboses and reflux, increases with age, when we look at individuals with possible venous problems, we have to remember that even very young people including teenagers can have severe venous disease.

Having now discussed the two major things that you definitely cannot change, your family history and your age, we are now going to move on to things that you can change, although in some cases this may be only be a little.

Obesity

There are some conflicting thoughts in the venous world about obesity. Of course, this is particularly relevant today, not only as we are seeing an epidemic of obesity in the Western world, but reports are suggesting many people are putting on weight during lockdown or in those people who are isolating.

A lot of people want obesity to be a risk factor for venous disease. There are a great many articles written about the "pressure" of fat in the pelvis and abdomen pushing on the veins, increasing the pressure and causing venous disease. In the grossly obese, there are also doctors and nurses that suggest that an overhanging belly can push on the thighs, further blocking the veins on sitting.

A recent major study looking at genetics, weight and venous disease also identified obesity as a risk factor for more severe venous disease.

However, it is highly likely that it is not quite as simple as this.

When we look at the distribution of people with varicose veins and hidden varicose veins, in other words venous reflux, there really is not much clear evidence that weight is a risk factor for developing venous reflux.

There is increasing evidence however that once you have venous reflux, the rate at which you deteriorate from simple varicose veins or hidden varicose veins through the swelling ankles, skin damage and eventually leg ulcers is much faster in those people who are obese than those people who are slim.

Indeed, there has been a recent study where patients with venous leg ulcers were encouraged to exercise, which not only improved their venous leg ulcers, but of course helped them lose weight. This really is not surprising when we know that treating varicose veins and stopping any venous reflux successfully cures leg ulcers, and we also understand that exercise increases the venous flow, reducing venous stasis.

Furthermore, some excellent work from a research department in Berlin has also shown that people who are quite sedentary during the day start developing tiny clots in the vein valves, even in healthy people, whereas those who walk several hours a day tend to have either very low numbers or even no sign of any such clots.

Therefore, putting all of the research together, it seems that obesity is not the problem, but is a sign of amount of exercise being taken.

The more patients exercise, the more they pump blood up their veins and the healthier their veins stay. This reduces the risks of any thromboses in any of the venous systems, and even if there is venous reflux, reduces the length of time that the venous blood refluxes and therefore also reduces venous stasis. Thus, even although venous reflux is still present, it is less likely to cause the complications of venous reflux disease.

The more exercise that a person does in a day, the slimmer they get and the less likely they are to be overweight or obese. Therefore, obesity seems to only be a marker of how much exercise is done. It appears to be that lack of exercise is the risk factor for both thrombotic venous disease or the deterioration of venous reflux disease, rather than obesity itself.

Flat feet and mobility issues

If you have read all of this book to this point, it will not surprise you at all that anything that affects the normal walking function will be detrimental to the venous system.

As we have seen previously, venous return to the heart needs the co-ordinated foot pump followed by calf pump and thigh pump to pump venous blood back to the heart from the legs.

Anything that interrupts this pumping, will be detrimental to the venous system. Reduced flow is more likely to lead to clots by Vichow's triad. Patients who have failed valves and venous reflux will have more time when the refluxing blood overloads the veins around the ankles, causing more inflammation and stasis. This is further worsened if the foot and leg pumps are inhibited.

Indeed, patients who have perfectly normal valves and no reflux can still get venous disease around their ankles and feet in the forms of swollen ankles and feet, skin changes such as venous eczema, red and brown stains and eventually venous leg ulcers, just because of the stasis. Therefore, although we have seen that valve failure causing venous reflux disease is the commonest cause of venous disease in the lower legs, stasis and obstruction can also cause these clinical changes.

It is beyond the scope of this book to go through all of the possible different mobility issues. Some are temporary, recovering from surgery, broken legs or other temporary mobility issues, and it is very important to follow physiotherapy advice during this recovery. In other cases, the lack of mobility is permanent and stable. In such cases, patients should work with their healthcare providers to reduce risks of venous disease using elevation of the legs, compression stockings, physiotherapy if relevant and machines that can help the veins pump externally. These can either work by stimulating the muscles to contract using electrical impulses or can actually pump blood by way of an inflatable bladder around the foot and/or leg.

Finally, a word about flat feet. There is quite a lot of research showing that people who have flat feet are more prone to having venous disease. This would not surprise anyone who has understood how the venous pumps work in the legs during walking. Making the foot pump less effective than normal, or even ineffective, has a massively detrimental effect on the venous flow back to the heart.

Of course, there are many different sorts of "flat feet", some curable and some not. Once again it is beyond the scope of this book to go through all of the different sorts of flat feet. However, if it is possible to use prosthetic implants to reconstruct the foot arch and to improve the foot function during walking, or even to potentially operate on the foot to restore the foot arch, then such methods would help restore the venous pump and reduce the risks of venous disease.

Previous venous disease

It will come as no surprise that previous venous disease is a risk factor for further venous disease in the future.

Looking at the clotting side first, people who have had previous venous thrombosis, such as deep vein thrombosis or superficial venous thrombosis, are more likely to have another one. If there is a very defined cause for the first thrombosis, such as major surgery followed by a full recovery to normal good health, then the risk might be low.

However, the propensity to get further venous thrombosis in the future is heightened with each episode that a person has previously had.

There has been some very interesting research which has suggested that if a person has one deep vein thrombosis, that is found quickly and treated aggressively so that it clears very quickly, it might be possible to end up with a completely normal deep vein that is still functioning normally once everything has settled down. This will be a surprise to many of the older doctors and nurses who have always been taught that once a person has had a deep vein thrombosis, it will destroy the deep veins and they will always have a problem in the future.

It turns out that people who end up with long-term problems with their deep veins are usually those who have more than one deep vein thrombosis, or a deep vein thrombosis that was not diagnosed quickly or not treated aggressively. The longer a deep vein thrombosis is sitting in the deep vein, or the more times a deep vein thrombosis has been sitting in the same place in the vein, the more inflammation it causes in the vein wall and the more scar tissue develops.

When deep vein thromboses have caused scar tissue in the deep veins, it has two main effects. The one that we used to think was most important was that the valves in the deep vein fail, causing deep vein incompetence or deep vein reflux. A great many doctors and nurses still think that this is the biggest problem in deep vein disease. A lot of effort has been put in to try and make a new valve for deep veins. As no such valve has ever been made to work reliably, most doctors and nurses still turn to compression as soon as they hear of deep vein disease.

However, most patients who have scarred deep veins actually have narrowing of the veins due to the scar tissue. This scar tissue causes an obstruction, preventing blood flowing out of the leg easily when pumped. Even although there is usualy reflux in the deep vein at the same time, the major problem appears to be this venous obstruction in the majority of patients.

This is good news because nowadays, if the obstruction is in a big vein in the pelvis or upper thigh, it is often possible to open the narrowing up using a balloon to dilate the vein, usually leaving a metal stent to keep the vein open.

When a patient has scarred deep veins and clinical problems, usually swollen ankle, discoloured lower leg and often accompanied by leg ulcers and pain on walking, the condition is called post-thrombotic syndrome (PTS). It can be a life changing event for the patient if this can be cured by the insertion of a stent to open up the obstruction. This has been one of the major recent advances in venous surgery and phlebology.

Patients who have had previous superficial venous thrombosis ("phlebitis") usually develop the problem as a complication of varicose veins. If the varicose veins have been treated adequately afterwards, this should reduce the risk of ever having superficial venous thrombosis again. Unfortunately, although doctors will help their patients through the acute pain of the superficial venous thrombosis, many fail to refer their patients to get their varicose veins treated. If the underlying cause of the thrombosis isn't removed, in this case the varicose veins, it is not surprising that it is highly likely that the problem will recur.

Moving on now to venous reflux disease, a previous history of varicose veins or hidden varicose veins will increase the risks of future venous problems. Obviously if a patient has had a problem due to venous reflux, such as a leg ulcer, venous eczema or a swollen ankle, and they have only been treated with compression or steroid creams, then naturally the problem will come back again. Simply if you do not treat the underlying venous reflux and have only done something temporary for the obvious symptoms or signs, then of course you haven't fixed anything, and the same problem will recur.

More distressing for many patients is the fact that many patients with varicose veins or hidden varicose veins will have already had venous surgery, and will think that they have been cured only to find that they get further venous problems in the future.

There are three reasons why varicose veins or hidden varicose veins can come back again after treatment:

1] the wrong vein was treated

2] the right vein was treated but with the wrong technique

3] veins that were originally normal have now lost their valves and become incompetent

Unfortunately, in non-specialist venous practices, the commonest cause of recurrence after venous surgery is the first of these reasons. When a patient has a very quick scan performed by someone who isn't doing complete venous scans regularly, they will only have the great saphenous vein and the small saphenous vein checked. Sometimes, patients are examined lying flat even though varicose veins do not show reflux in that position!

Because there is virtually no quality assurance currently in venous surgery, nobody is checking the quality of such scans and so patients are left to decide for themselves whether they trust the investigations that they have had. Most patients do not delve too deeply into the backgrounds of their doctor, and most patients trust doctors as professionals to do their very best.

Unfortunately, although doctors may try their very best, not all doctors specialise in veins nor set up their practice to provide the best care. This is one of the reasons we have set up the College of Phlebology Venous Registry which tracks patients over the years, allowing patients to feedback every year as to whether their treatment was successful or not. Over the years, doctors, clinics and hospitals getting good results will be differentiated from those who do not.

However, in the meantime, patients should expect that when they are having a varicose vein scan, they should be standing upright or lying on a tilt table that is virtually upright, to look for reflux due to gravity. All of the veins in the legs should be scanned and this rarely takes less than 15 minutes per leg as a minimum. Scans that take less time than this are unlikely to be checking all of the possible sources of venous reflux.

If a doctor finds one vein refluxing, and decides only to treat that, and does not look for any other sources of reflux, then it is not surprising that their patients will have a much higher chance of recurrence. Often doctors will find major reflux in a saphenous vein and not look for pelvic vein reflux or incompetent perforator vein reflux as well. This is what we mean by saying "the wrong vein was treated".

One of the biggest problems we have identified over the last 20 years in most venous practices, is that we have found that 1 in 6 women who have varicose veins of the legs have got a major contribution of their venous reflux coming from pelvic varicose veins. These varicose veins emerge from around the vulva, perineum or buttocks, refluxing blood into the leg varicose veins.

Often these can be seen but sometimes they are not visible. Interestingly, this is also found in 1 in 30 men with leg varicose veins.

However, very few doctors who treat varicose veins look for varicose veins emerging from the pelvis, never mind offering treatment. Hence 1 in 6 women undergoing varicose vein surgery in most practices will not have all of their refluxing veins treated and therefore, will have a higher chance of getting their varicose veins back again sometime in the future.

The second commonest cause of recurrence after surgery for venous reflux is that the right veins were treated but using the wrong techniques. This can be as simple as doctors who still strip veins, even though published research has shown a high risk of veins growing back again after stripping. When veins grow back again after stripping, they never develop new valves and so they are always incompetent.

Other patients think that they have had the latest techniques but, just like every technique, to be successful it has to be used appropriately. Many patients have endovenous laser or radiofrequency, thinking that because they have the latest minimally invasive techniques the operation will be successful.

Unfortunately, veins vary in size and shape, and a great many non-specialists use standard settings when treating patients. Not surprisingly, veins that are larger need more energy to have the same effect as normal veins, and veins that are smaller need less energy to have the same effect. What makes it even more difficult is that it is not just the size of the vein but the thickness of the vein wall.

In our clinics we see large numbers of patients who have had previous endovenous surgery elsewhere and are convinced that their main veins have been treated. Hence, they are understandably concerned as to why they have developed recurrent varicose veins. Sometimes, when we scan the patients, we cannot find any evidence the target vein was treated at all. This usually happens when a low power is used causing a thrombosis in the short-term, temporarily blocking the vein and making the varicose veins disappear. As the vein itself has not been destroyed, the thrombus then slowly dissolves away, allowing the reflux to return and the varicose veins to re-appear.

In addition, there has been a fad for the last 15 years or so to use foam sclerotherapy in N2 truncal veins as well as the more superficial N3 veins under the skin. Many doctors will tell their patients that this is cheaper and quicker, and indeed there has been a lot of publicity in the press claiming that you can cure all of the varicose veins with one injection!

Unfortunately, research has shown that foam sclerotherapy is not anywhere near as effective as using heat such as endovenous laser or radiofrequency in the larger and thicker walled N2 truncal veins. Once again, patients are initially happy because the foam sclerotherapy has caused a thrombosis that blocks the incompetent truncal vein and so they feel that they have improved. However, clinical research studies have shown that a large proportion then go on to re-open again and venous reflux recurs in the same vein that was previously treated.

Proponents of foam sclerotherapy will say that it is easy to keep re-treating the veins, but of course most patients want to have a treatment that works in the long term and not keep going back for top ups. In addition, each time a new procedure is performed there are the usual inherent risks of the procedure.

As such, these are typical examples of the right vein being identified for treatment but then the wrong technique being used allowing the same veins to recur with recurrent reflux in the future.

Finally, the third risk of getting varicose veins or hidden varicose veins back again after treatment, is the risk of veins that were competent at the time of the initial treatment becoming incompetent in the future.

This is called "de-novo reflux" or "new reflux". It is a bit like going to a dentist and having a cavity filled, and then getting another cavity in another tooth later on. It is not that the treatment failed, it is just that there was a progression of the disease. This is the same argument as we find in de novo reflux.

As such, if a patient has the right veins treated with the right techniques, and then gets new reflux in a vein that was previously found to be competent, it would not have been possible to have stopped this at the original operation. It is merely disease progression in a previously normal vein.

You might ask how we can tell whether such reflux is truly "de novo reflux" or whether the original scan was wrong. This is the importance of the College of Phlebology Venous Registry. The proportion of treated patients coming back with recurrent varicose veins every year from each doctor, can indicate whether their recurrence is "de novo" or not.

We know from previous studies that the risk of someone who comes from a family that has a high prevalence of varicose veins, but who does not have varicose veins themselves at the time, will have a 3.0-4.5% chance per year of developing "de novo" varicose veins. Therefore, the natural deterioration of a person with a familial propensity of getting varicose veins, actually developing them is 3.0-4.5% chance per year.

Over the last 20 years we have continued to audit our practice in my clinic, and in the long term have found that our recurrence rate after treatment is 3.3% per year. This means that by using The Whiteley Protocol®, we have eliminated the chance of treating the wrong vein, or using the wrong technique, and we are now only seeing "de novo" recurrence in our patients returning with any recurrent varicose veins. To my knowledge we are the only clinic in the world that has managed to show this in the long term.

Although in the past it has taken us a lot of time and effort to do these audits, the new College of Phlebology Venous Registry will do this easily. It will monitor all patients attending any participating doctor or clinic. Over the years, patients will be able to be certain that their doctors are maintaining excellent results. Any doctors who do not maintain low recurrence rates will be notified and either re-trained or lose the accreditation of the registry. Therefore, patients will be able to choose their doctors through the registry, confident that their doctor is being monitored and all of their results checked.

Cancer

Over the last decade it has become increasingly well known that having a malignancy increases the risks of venous thrombosis. This is not simply because the tumour is pushing on the veins, although in rare situations this can be the case. It is a complication that is not really understood.

It must be due to something changing in the blood but so far, no one has been able to identify with certainty what the factor or factors are.

It is interesting that up to about 10 years ago, patients who developed an unexpected deep vein thrombosis had their blood screened for a thrombophilia as one of the first tests. Now, patients who develop an unexpected deep vein thrombosis, particularly if they are over 40 years old, are screened for an undiagnosed cancer.

Anyone who starts developing unexpected deep vein thromboses or superficial venous thromboses should undergo a series of tests looking for hidden cancers. Typically this would include a chest x-ray, mammogram for females, blood tests for tumour markers, scans of the liver, pancreas and ovaries (in women) and possibly a colonoscopy to check for bowel tumours.

Patients with cancer who are in a lockdown or who are isolating, are more likely to get a deep vein thrombosis or superficial venous thrombosis. People who develop an unexpected deep vein thrombosis or superficial venous thrombosis should be checked for an undiagnosed or hidden cancer if they are not aware they have one.

Recent surgery

Nowadays we tend to think that we can bounce back after surgery very quickly. Increasing medical technology, minimally invasive surgery, better painkillers, and early mobilisation have all helped us get back to normal life quicker than ever before in medical history.

Unfortunately though, our bodies have not evolved at the same rate. At the end of the day, the process by which we heal, initially by inflammation, followed by regeneration of tissues, and modification of scar tissue, still takes time. Many people know that after even quite minor surgery affecting the abdomen or pelvis, they feel very "under the weather" for 2-6 weeks. This is the body's natural response to trauma.

If an animal is injured, a combination of hormones and brain function will make them feel depressed and they will crawl into a cave or basket to recover. This gives the body chance to put all of the available energy into healing. Once the body is starting to heal, the patient suddenly starts to feel better again and wants to get back to normal life and mobility.

This is a natural process that should be understood. Anyone undergoing surgery and then going home will often feel like curling up in front of the TV or staying in bed for 2-4 weeks at least, while their body recovers. Although this is very good from a healing point of view, unfortunately it does increase the risk of deep vein thrombosis or superficial venous thrombosis.

This is why following any surgery, particularly any abdominal surgery, physiotherapists will recommend exercises, compression stockings will be recommended and high-risk patients will be given heparin injections daily for a week or two whilst still at risk. All of these interventions are aimed at reducing the risks of developing venous thromboses during the post-operative period.

We have now gone through most of the major risks for venous disease, which may well help identify whether you or members of your family or friends might be more at risk of developing a venous problem during a lockdown or isolation period.

We are now going to look more specifically at what you can do at home to try and prevent a venous problem during a lockdown or period of isolation.

Chapter 6

What you can do at home

Although venous disease is very common, and can have very severe complications, it is one of the medical conditions that you can do a lot yourself to avoid getting problems.

There are some instances, particularly if a complication has occurred, where you will need medical help. In the next chapter we are going to start looking at specific conditions you may notice and will give advice as to what you should do, and how urgently.

However, this chapter is going to look at things you can do yourself at home to try and avoid complications of venous disease, and if you have underlying venous problems, how to reduce the risk of deterioration or complications.

By understanding the previous chapters and understanding both how the venous system works and what can go wrong with it, a lot of the following points should make perfect sense.

Exercise

You will not be surprised that the first thing I have written about to prevent complications of venous disease and to reduce any deterioration is exercise. However not all exercise is equal. Understanding the benefits of different exercises will also help you choose the right regime for yourself.

There are two main reasons to exercise to keep your veins healthy.

The first is related to the veins and is to keep the flow of blood from the feet, up through the legs and into the heart as fast as possible. Lying down and elevating the legs above the level of the heart will allow blood to flow back to the heart without a problem, due to changing the pressure. However, it won't actually increase the flow to levels where you get the benefits of reducing thromboses (clots in the veins) and developing the wall shear stress that keeps the veins healthy.

The second is to reduce the risk of putting on weight and obesity. As we discussed earlier, weight by itself probably doesn't actually cause venous problems. However, if you are putting on weight it is a pretty good sign that you are not getting enough exercise and that you are at risk of getting increased complications from venous disease. As we have discussed, this might mean clots in the leg veins, either deep or superficial, or if you have venous reflux, increased levels of stasis around the ankles and deterioration of symptoms and signs in the legs.

Different people have different preferences for exercise and of course, during a lockdown or isolation, have different surroundings and therefore different opportunities for exercise.

Fortunately, the best exercise for veins is walking. As we discussed previously, walking normally coordinates the venous pumps in the leg starting with the foot pump, pumping blood into the calf, then the calf pump, pumping blood into the thigh and finally the thigh pump, pumping blood up into the pelvis towards the heart. When the muscles relax, blood starts to fall backwards towards the foot. Provided all of the valves are working, there should not be any venous reflux in the leg veins.

If you do have valve failure and reflux, you will get venous reflux in the leg veins. However, by walking, you are reducing the static pressure at the ankle and are reducing venous stasis. Both of these factors reduce the damage caused by venous reflux.

Hence walking, or any other exercise that mimics walking, such as treadmill walking, jogging, running or using a cross trainer is probably the best exercise you can do for your vein health.

Many people like cycling or rowing as these can be done either on machines at home or if you are lucky enough, to cycle on the road or row on a local river or canal. Although these are good cardiovascular exercises, they do not seem to have the same benefits for leg veins as they do not have a coordinated pump action from feet to heart.

Cycling in particular is a very interesting exercise for a vein surgeon. Although cyclists clearly use a lot of calories, there are some potential problems with cycling as an exercise for veins. Depending on how the foot and the pedal is used, the foot pump may not be activated as part of the activity. The coordination of the pumps is not the same as in normal walking or running. The pressures developed in the calf muscles are very high and it is possible that such high pressures might increase the risk of perforating vein reflux. Indeed, I have published a case report where vigorous cycling clearly caused valve failure in one perforator and an overlying varicose vein to appear.

Finally, some patients can have an anatomical abnormality where there is compression of the veins and potentially arteries behind the knee or in the groin, entrapping the vessels and potentially causing clots. In the venous system, this has been described although it is very rare to actually cause venous thrombosis. However, we do not know how many patients have lower levels of venous outflow obstruction from this compression, but do not get bad enough to actually thrombose the vein.

Without doubt these exercises are better than doing nothing but are probably not as good for the veins as walking. I hope that we will be able to continue our research into the effects of cycling and other activities on the veins to elucidate the facts further in the future.

Finally, some people live in flats or houses and either cannot or do not want to leave at all. For those staying indoors all of the time, benefit can be obtained from walking exercises using treadmills, walking up and down stairs or even walking on the spot. Therefore, you can get all of the health benefits of exercise very cheaply and in very limited space.

Diet

There is a massive obsession at the moment with diets, nutrition and nutritional supplements for all sorts of healthcare.

However, there is precious little evidence that any of this has much effect on veins, vein health or the venous circulation.

Hence for patients with no known venous disease, diet or supplements probably has very little to offer over and above sensible advice on good diets.

Without doubt, good advice would be to have a balanced diet with good nutrition and vitamins. Furthermore, a diet that keeps your weight stable with a BMI that is as close to normal as possible (remembering that if you are muscular you should probably have a higher BMI than is noted as "normal") is probably optimal.

For patients who have venous disease, or symptoms of aching in the legs secondary to venous disease, then there has been some research to show that flavonoids - or more particularly micronized purified flavonoid fraction (MPFF) - can be beneficial. Research has shown a reduction in discomfort and, at the cellular level, the glycocaylix on the endothelial cell that can become thinned in venous disease, is largely reconstituted in patients taking MPFF.

Another remedy that has been used with venous disease is horse chestnut (which the active ingredient is Escin). This appears to have some effect of reducing inflammation, oedema (swelling) and therefore discomfort in patients with venous disease.

There are a great many other supplements as well, but the effect of diets and supplements in venous disease is really quite small.

However, patients who have venous leg ulcers do have a different problem. When there is an open sore such as a venous leg ulcer, and the body is continually trying to repair it, the body uses a lot of Vitamin C and protein. Vitamin C is absolutely essential in wound healing, and it is well known that vitamin C deficiency (scurvy) causes well healed wounds to re-open again.

Research on patients with venous leg ulcers has shown that the majority have very low levels of vitamin C. In addition, continually producing new cells, and secreting protein rich fluid to try and form scabs and help skin to grow back over the wound, means the body loses a lot of protein.

Therefore, patients with venous leg ulcers should take vitamin C supplements daily and have high protein diets.

Hydration

Hydration is a very interesting subject. All medical students are taught that a normal person needs 1.5 L a day. Indeed, if you are admitted to hospital and are not able to eat or drink, you will be given intravenous fluids by a drip. Unless you are losing fluid or have another problem, you will be maintained on exactly 1.5 L per day.

However, for some reason, health websites, magazines, beauticians, personal trainers and a whole host of other para-medical people give the most amazing advice suggesting that it is "healthy" to drink 2 L of water a day - and sometimes more. I have even seen quotes of 3 L a day, particularly on websites selling water. The way this advice is given often gives the impression that this is two or more litres of water needed in addition to all the other food and fluids you drink in a day!

Therefore, you need to think very carefully about what is meant by hydration and how much water you actually need. Firstly, you must remember that when you eat food, there is a lot of water hidden in it. Not only things like salad and other fruit and vegetables that clearly have water in them, and of course soups, but carbohydrate breaks down to carbon dioxide and water in your cells. Therefore, if you are eating a normal diet, you are getting about half a litre of water per day hidden in the food.

When you then drink fruit juices, tea, coffee, wine or beer, you are having even more fluid.

Now, you then have to think about losses. If your tea or coffee has caffeine in it, this acts as a diuretic, making you pass more urine and so therefore you might end up a bit more dehydrated even if you are drinking higher volumes. Similarly, alcoholic drinks also have a diuretic effect dehydrating you even though you are drinking fluid.

In addition, if you turn your heating up, or do a lot of exercise, or have a temperature, you may be losing more fluid across your skin then you think. You lose fluid from the skin by evaporation, not only by sweating. Therefore, rather than generally thinking you have to drink a certain amount of water, it is better to realise that you are an individual and you need to decide on how much water you should be drinking yourself.

The simplest way of doing this is to follow two simple rules.

Firstly, drink water when you are thirsty.

Secondly, your urine should be a very light straw coloured yellow. If your urine is completely colourless, you are probably drinking too much fluid. If your urine is dark and smelly, then you are probably drinking too little fluid. The reason for this is that most people produce the same amount of urea every day. This urea is the yellow colour in urine. If you are producing the same amount of this yellow colour, then the more water you are drinking, the more diluted it is and the lighter the yellow. If you are drinking so much that you cannot even see a yellow colour, you are probably overhydrated. If you drink too little, the yellow colour gets darker as the urea gets more concentrated.

However, if you eat a lot of protein, you produce more urea and so this makes the urine monitoring much more difficult.

Following the simple rules of drinking when you are thirsty and keeping your urine straw coloured are likely to keep you very healthy and normally hydrated. This only becomes a problem if you have a medical problem with liver or kidneys, are taking drugs that can affect urine output such as diuretics, or if you eat lots of protein.

Finally, as far as veins are concerned, being slightly over hydrated is not a problem. What you want to avoid is being dehydrated. As we saw before with Virchow's triad, dehydration can lead to an increased risk of venous thrombosis and must be avoided. On the other hand, it is not sensible to massively overhydrate as there is a condition called "water intoxication".

People who keep drinking water all the time can end up with very low blood salts, resulting in an increase of oedema (fluid) in the brain. This clouds the thinking and can make people irritable. Although it is not common to have severe water intoxication, I have seen a patient with this. She bought a 2 litre bottle of water into the consultation with her, and had a sip every minute or two throughout the consultation.

Therefore, although it is better to be a little overhydrated than underhydrated, getting addicted to drinking water or making regular drinking habitual even when you are not thirsty, is not a good idea.

Of course, all of this advice is relevant for those people who are fit and healthy at home during lockdown or who are in isolation. Things change if a patient has a fever, in which case the temperature goes up, their water losses go up and quite often they do not feel well enough to drink water. In these cases, keeping the patient hydrated is essential.

Once again however, monitoring the colour of the urine is a very sensible way to know the level of hydration.

Compression stockings

Compression socks, stockings and tights come in a great range of different makes and styles.

Before we look at the different sorts of compression stockings and where you might get them, it's useful to know how they work, what they are useful for and what they are not useful for.

From the discussion earlier in this book about the venous circulation, we saw how the arterial blood is pumped from the heart down to the feet through the arteries at high pressure. Once the blood has gone through the capillaries, given up the oxygen and nutrients and picked up the carbon dioxide and waste products, it emerges into the veins with very little pressure. It is only the venous pumps in the foot, calf and thigh that are activated during movement that can pump the blood back to the heart, provided the valves are also working.

Many people are now much less mobile than they have been previously. This might be due to working from home or being stuck at home looking after children or doing other things, particularly if forced to during a lockdown or isolation. Reducing the amount of activity means that the blood flow out of the veins in the lower leg, ankle and foot reduces. If severe, this can lead to venous stasis. Stasis can happen in patients with normal veins but is even worse in people who have venous reflux (varicose veins or hidden varicose veins).

In the simplest form, in a stationary person the pressure of blood is the column of blood measured from the heart vertically downwards to the foot. This is the "static" pressure of blood in a column. Therefore, when you are standing still, the pressure at the ankle is maximal. When you are sitting, the pressure is less but still significant. This pressure can be reduced by movement, as movement pumps the blood up the leg, stopping the static pressure of the column. The pressure only disappears when the ankle is brought up to the same level as the heart, and there is no vertical difference between the two.

As we have pointed out several times during this book, exercises using the foot and leg muscle pumps are optimal to return venous blood towards the heart. However, many people are not able to exercise as much as they would like. A compression stocking will have several advantages in such patients.

Firstly, the simple increase in pressure around the ankle changes the pressure gradient between heart and ankle. This means that the column of blood that lies vertically from your heart to ankle is pushing against the vein walls with the pressure equal to the height of that column of blood. If you're wearing compression stockings, then the amount of pressure pushing on the outside of the leg, transmitted through to the veins, goes some way to countering that pressure. Hence, we are reducing the venous pressure on the vein wall by the amount of pressure that the compression stocking generates.

Secondly, the pressure on the tissue and veins in the AC3 - i.e. the compartment just under the skin where the subcutaneous fat and most superficial veins lie - gives a very beneficial effect to the wearer of the stockings. In these superficial veins, the veins are somewhat compressed, meaning that blood flows faster through the veins. This increased flow reduces the risk of clotting (venous thrombosis).

In addition, any venous stasis is also reduced. If there are any veins that are full of blood that is not moving significantly, the compression reduces this reservoir, reducing the volume of venous stasis. As we saw previously, venous stasis causes inflammation of the veins and surrounding tissues. Reduction of the amount of venous stasis therefore reduces this inflammation.

Finally, any fluid collecting outside of the veins in the tissue (called oedema) is also encouraged back into the veins by the compression pressure of the stocking.

Hence the effect of properly fitted compression stockings is a reduction of risk of deep vein thrombosis and superficial venous thrombosis, a reduction of stasis and inflammation at the ankle making the leg feel better as well as actively reducing damage due to chronic inflammation, and also a reduction of swelling of the ankle by reducing the oedema.

Now we can turn to what stockings are actually available.

Some of these are medical grade, and give quite specific amounts of compression, maximal around the foot and ankle and decreasing up the leg (called graduated pressure). The medical compression garments have different grades of compression depending how much compression is required, usually ranging from 1 to 4 although there are two different grading systems that are used regularly.

The stockings that are used in hospitals to reduce the risk of deep vein thrombosis are usually called anti-thromboembolic disease stockings or "TED" stockings and these tend to be of lower compression and much lighter material.

Many fashion stockings now include some compression to try and give a little bit of support and make the legs feel better, although the amounts of compression are usually much lower than the lowest medical class.

Everybody has a different shape leg and so manufacturers produce a range of compression stockings to try and get as close as possible to the compression that you need. However, it is quite likely that your leg will not be exactly the same as one of their standard shapes, and so even with careful measuring, sometimes you have to try several different makes or sizes to find one that fits you comfortably.

There are now some very helpful websites and companies that will aid you to measure your own compression stockings and deliver them to your door. In addition, nurses at family doctors' surgeries, hospitals or clinics will often be able to measure you and order appropriate stockings, and a lot of pharmacies also supply this service.

Machines to help venous circulation

It is also possible to purchase a wide range of machines or gadgets to be used at home to help the venous circulation.

Many of these were developed over a decade ago, to reduce the risk of deep vein thrombosis on a flight when the idea of "economy class syndrome" was first conceived. However, many are still available.

Some of the simplest are devices such as airbags, hinged pedals or things that you roll with your feet, all of which encourage you to move your ankle and feet in a repetitive motion, to increase the foot pump and the calf pump.

There are some other more expensive devices that stimulate the muscles in the lower leg, causing twitches which helps blood to be pumped back up the veins by muscle contraction. One or two combine such electronic stimulation along with a rocking motion for you to do actively.

We performed some research on several of these devices many years ago. The good news is that any of them that make your ankle joint move, have some effect on pumping the blood back up the veins and are therefore beneficial. As a general rule, the more the ankle joint moves, the more effective the pumping action on the venous blood.

Of course, with the ones that stimulate the muscles, it is harder to know this for sure without doing research scans, as the effectiveness does not rely on the movement of the ankle joint but muscle twitching caused by electronic impulses.

Finally, there are also some devices that rhythmically inflate and deflate air bladders that can be fitted around the foot or lower legs. These compress the feet and lower legs, helping pump venous blood back to the heart.

Most healthy people probably do not need any of these additional machines, unless they are stuck for long periods of time in front of a desk. In such cases, they may find compression stockings or the mechanical machines useful.

People who have poor mobility, or who are unable to stand easily to exercise by themselves, may find huge benefit from these machines with or without compression stockings.

Pregnancy

Although this does not fit easily in any particular section, it is worth discussing what someone who is pregnant might do to try and reduce the risk of venous problems while stuck at home during a lockdown or isolation.

Generally, early pregnancy in the first 3-6 months, has little effect on the venous system. Unless a person has previous venous problems before getting pregnant, there is nothing particularly to watch out for in this time period, over and above the general advice given previously. Some patients who had varicose veins before pregnancy and did not have them treated before they got pregnant, will start getting more uncomfortable. Although the previous advice has always been to leave varicose veins until after a person has finished all of her children, this was because the old sort of surgery was unsuccessful and varicose veins usually recurred.

The new advice, from units such as our own with very low recurrence rates, is to get the veins treated as soon as you know that you have them. This means that subsequent pregnancies will be a lot more comfortable and have a much reduced risk of superficial venous thrombosis ("phlebitis"). However, no one is going to perform venous surgery on a pregnant lady, and therefore I'm afraid the only option is compression stockings and walking until after birth. Three months after birth, when everything has returned to normal, is the optimum time to get the veins treated.

In the last trimester of pregnancy, 7-9 months, the abdomen swells considerably as the foetus grows rapidly. In addition, a mother increases her blood volume from 5 L to 7 L - an increase of 40%. Women with pelvic varicose veins, also known as pelvic congestion syndrome, will often start seeing swollen varicose veins of the vulva and vagina. These are often associated with haemorrhoids.

Unfortunately, although the symptoms are likely to be far worse and the veins far bigger, just as with the previous months, there is no specific advice that can be given apart from wearing compression stockings. Companies now make specific maternity compression tights which have a panel to allow expansion of the pregnant abdomen to the front. Compression stockings at this stage will not only improve the symptoms but will also reduce the risk of any superficial venous thrombosis in any large varicose veins appearing on the surface.

As before, the most important thing for the future is to make sure that as soon as the baby is born and things are returning to normal, you have the veins investigated and treated to reduce the risks of any repetition in subsequent pregnancies.

Misinformation and scams

Finally for this section about what you can do at home to keep your veins healthy and to know what vein problems you can solve by yourself, is to be very sceptical about "miracle cures" and "cheap treatments" that you will see promoted widely, particularly on the Internet.

With regard to the "miracle cures" that can be posted to you, these come in a whole lot of formats from supplements, diets as well as products.

We have already gone through what goes wrong with veins and you can see that most of it is quite logical. A normal healthy person who is exercising is at a very low risk of getting blood clots. If you have venous reflux disease because your valves have failed, there is nothing that you can do to cure this apart from having a proper colour flow duplex ultrasound scan and having appropriate surgery. Of course, you can reduce any deterioration until surgery by walking regularly.

The products that do have some evidence that they help have been quoted already in this book, and particularly this chapter. Anything that keeps your legs moving and the venous blood being pumped up the veins, will reduce the risk of clots and will also slow down the deterioration and reduce the complications of venous reflux disease. The few supplements that have shown to have some effect at being anti-inflammatory, reducing oedema and discomfort are only useful for symptomatic relief and do not get to the bottom of the problem. Therefore, if you do spend money on these, don't expect that they will get rid of the problem completely. They merely help symptoms in the short term.

Any drug, alternative medicine or supplement that is shown to have any real effect is usually made prescription only and has severe warnings attached to it. For instance, when St John's Wort was shown to interact with warfarin and decrease the effectiveness of the blood thinning effects of warfarin, increasing the risk of thromboses, a great amount of publicity was made about this and warnings have now been placed on the Internet and on responsible packaging.

There are also many very weird ideas such as leeches or yoga for varicose veins, none of which actually have any real or lasting effect. You would be able to know this yourself if you have read through the logic in this book. As we have seen, most venous surgery is about physical movement and whether blood flow is fast or stopped from refluxing through damaged valves. None of this is affected by leeches or static poses in yoga, nor of course by dietary supplements.

When it comes to treating venous conditions, we have already touched upon the requirement for expert scanning of the veins to find all of the sources of problems, and then a research led approach to correcting all of the areas where flow is abnormal in the leg veins. Merely setting up a cheap clinic where a doctor does a quick scan with a cheap scanner, and says that they use the latest equipment, may well keep prices down, but is highly unlikely to give the results that you will want in the medium to long term.

Good medicine is rarely effective as cutting corners usually means cutting quality somewhere along the line. Commercial entities will try to persuade you that they can do the same job cheaper than research led clinics such as our own. When such services and their doctors have joined the College of Phlebology Venous Registry and their results are available for all to see after two or three years, then they will be able to justify such a claim. However, research and logic from those of us who understand the science of veins and vein treatments make such an outcome highly unlikely.

There is a reason that there are so many sayings along the lines of "a fool and their money are often parted" and "buy cheap, buy twice". Unfortunately, for some reason, many people think that these simple human traits do not extend into medicine. They do and so you should be very careful as to what you spend your money on or consent to have done to you.

We are now going to go through venous conditions, explaining which ones need to be treated urgently in a specialist vein centre, those that need to be treated but not urgently and those that you can treat at home. I will explain the science behind each one so that putting this explanation together with all you have read so far, you should be able to make a good decision as to what to do if you or anyone around you develops any of these conditions.

Chapter 7

Treatments for venous conditions and medical versus cosmetic

In Chapter 2, we discussed the symptoms and signs that you might notice if you have clinically significant venous disease or have developed a complication due to venous disease. We concentrated on what you would feel or see, to help direct you to thinking about what the underlying cause might be.

In this chapter, we are going to think about the underlying cause. As doctors, we need to know the underlying cause for any symptoms or signs, as this determines how we treat you. Hence patients turning up with completely different symptoms or signs might end up having very similar treatments if the underlying cause is the same. Conversely other patients presenting with very similar external signs, might have completely different underlying causes for these signs and therefore need completely different treatments.

For example, one person with aching varicose veins on their calves, and another patient with a venous leg ulcer, appear to have completely different conditions. However, both can be due to valves failing in the great saphenous vein and three incompetent perforators in the lower leg. Both will have successful treatment if they have the great saphenous vein and all three incompetent perforators treated, stopping the reflux. This will stop the aching varicose veins in the first patient, and in the second patient the venous ulcer will completely heal and disappear. Therefore, what appears to be two completely separate conditions at presentation actually has the same underlying cause in each, and the treatment for both is the same.

Conversely, two patients might both turn up with red, hot, tender and swollen lumps on their legs that suddenly appeared. Both will have "phlebitis" or as we have seen, a superficial venous thrombosis. However, on colour flow duplex ultrasound scanning we may find that the first merely has one vein just under the skin in the AC3 that has thrombosed with no other underlying cause, whereas the other may have thrombosis extending from this superficial N3 vein in the AC3, down into the truncal N2 vein, and encroaching close to the deep-vein (N1 vein).

The former patient can be treated safely with non-steroidal anti-inflammatory (aspirin or similar tablets or gel) and medical compression stockings. However, the second patient is at risk of a pulmonary embolism and therefore the treatment is full anticoagulation, and then when resolved, endovenous ablation of the truncal N2 vein to stop it ever happening again. Hence despite both presenting with a very similar symptom and sign, treatment ends up being completely different.

This is one of the reasons why it is foolhardy for any doctor or nurse to give advice to a patient with suspected venous disease without having a good quality and high resolution colour flow duplex ultrasound scan, that has been performed by an expert in venous duplex ultrasonography. It is only with that test as a minimum, that doctors and nurses know the underlying cause for any symptoms or signs and can start planning the optimal treatment. In some cases, other tests are needed, but fortunately in the majority of cases, this one diagnostic test is sufficient.

Having explained this, we will now go through the venous diseases that are usually found.

Varicose veins and hidden varicose veins

For thousands of years, names in medicine were quite simple. Doctors described what they could see, smell or feel and make diagnoses on these findings. There were very few tests that could be done and so everything was done with the hands, eyes, nose and sometimes tastebuds. Nowadays we would call this a "clinical" diagnosis, meaning without tests.

In the 1890s, the advent of x-rays started allowing doctors to look inside the body and understand what was going on deep inside, that might cause the symptoms and signs that they were picking up clinically. Over the next hundred years or so, there has been an explosion of diagnostic tests including blood tests, urine tests, ultrasound, CT scanning, MRI, PET scans, radioisotope scans and so on, that have allowed doctors not only to diagnose patients much more accurately, but also to understand how certain conditions or diseases develop.

Of course we still do not know everything, and this is why those of us involved in research are still pushing the boundaries in our areas, writing papers, presenting research, attending conferences and editing journals, so we can keep finding out the latest ideas in our area, to continually improve our understanding of the disease and hence our treatment of patients. Those who are not actively involved in research tend to get the information after many years, when the research is embodied into teaching or new devices and this then reaches the majority of doctors.

Most diseases and conditions were named historically, before we had the tests to help us with the understanding as to why the condition was occurring.

Varicose veins is an excellent example of this. I will now explain this by going through some of the recent history of varicose veins.

The first known description of varicose veins that was written down was approximately 2600 years ago (600 BC) by an Indian doctor called Rishi Sushruta. As most people would understand today, varicose veins were described as abnormally bulging veins on the legs on standing that disappeared on lying flat. Even in Roman times, such veins were often hooked out to remove them.

However it wasn't until the end of the 1800s that a doctor called Trendelenburg studied some post-mortem specimens and found that people who had varicose veins in the lower legs, had valves that were not working in the truncal veins higher up in the legs and groin. He therefore proposed that we should tie the truncal vein (the great saphenous vein), in order to stop the blood falling down the vein because the valves were not working. This was the first understanding that the bulging veins were caused by valves that were not working in the underlying veins, and therefore the blood was refluxing the wrong way down the veins on standing. He was the first to suggest that stopping this reflux would cure varicose veins, although initially he suggested to tie the great saphenous vein in the mid-thigh, rather than in the groin.

In the 1950s, the Doppler ultrasound was invented. This allowed doctors to beam ultrasound energy into the body at different points, and then listen for any of the ultrasound that was bounced back from inside the body. The Doppler ultrasound machine compared the frequency of the returning reflections with the initial frequency passed into the body. If anything was moving significantly inside the body, the frequency was changed by that movement. This is called the "Doppler shift". It is beyond the scope of this book to go further into this phenomena, but all that is important for this book is that you understand it is possible to measure blood that is moving deep inside the body, using ultrasound alone.

Over the 1970s and through to the 1990s, companies started putting normal ultrasound (called "greyscale" or "B mode" ultrasound) which gave black-and-white images made up of reflections from structures inside the body, together with the Doppler ultrasound which showed movement. By using clever and very fast computers, the blood cells that are moving can be given a colour, usually red or blue, whereas everything that is not moving is kept black and white. In this way we can see blood flowing in the arteries and veins by colour, superimposed onto a whole picture of that section of the body. This means we can see skin, fat, muscle, arteries, veins and nerves, and can also see the blood flowing inside the arteries and veins.

We now call this combination the "colour flow duplex ultrasound" although some scientists and authors will call it "colour flow Doppler", "colour coded duplex", "triplex", "venous duplex ultrasound" or a host of similar names.

As the technology has increased, this is now incredibly accurate and we can even see valves if we need to. In addition, we can see blood clots (thrombus) inside the veins as well as compressions on the outside of the vessel.

Another nice thing about the colour flow Doppler in these colour flow duplex ultrasound machines is that we can see which direction the blood is flowing. Therefore, when a patient is standing upright, and the calf is squeezed, blood is seen to flow up the veins in the legs from the calf pump.

When pressure is released on the calf, blood starts to fall back down the leg veins but stops within half a second as all of the valves close. Of course, in patients whose valves have failed, this venous blood will continue to reflux back down the vein. This is very obvious on colour flow duplex ultrasound. This is the way we can diagnose venous reflux non-invasively.

By using different techniques, we can also see reflux in pelvic veins and perforating veins, allowing us to get a complete diagnosis of venous reflux.

As we can see the veins very well, if blood is not flowing in the veins at all due to thrombus, the thrombus can be seen as well as the lack of flow in that area. We are able to differentiate between a completely occluded and a partially occluded vein, where a thrombus is seen attached to the vein wall, with blood flow passing around it on one side.

When we are looking for venous reflux, we need to use gravity and so patients are standing up or lying at quite a sharp angle close to standing up. When we are looking for clots, we can lie patients flat.

The reason I have explained all of this is that you will now understand that although patients, doctors and nurses can see varicose veins that bulge in the legs on standing, it is only when a colour flow duplex ultrasound scan is performed that we can find which vein, or combination of veins, are refluxing and causing the problem. Absolutely no doctor or nurse in the world will be able to tell you with any certainty what the cause of any varicose veins is without performing a colour flow duplex ultrasound scan first.

There is also a second reason to explain this in such detail. This is how we diagnose the hidden varicose veins that we have talked about previously in this book.

As we have noted previously, some 15-20% of adults have varicose veins visible on standing in the legs, When we do population studies with colour flow duplex ultrasound scan, we find approximately 30-40% of adults have venous reflux in their superficial (N2, N3 or perforating) veins in the legs. Thus 15-20% of the adult population have hidden varicose veins.

You might think that hidden varicose veins don't matter if they do not cause any bulging varicose veins on the surface. However, this is not the case. In the early 1990s, ground-breaking research showed that at least half of the patients with venous leg ulcers had "hidden varicose veins". Before that research, it was commonly assumed that patients with venous leg ulcers had deep vein reflux (reflux in the N1 veins) that could not be treated surgically. This is why all patients with venous leg ulcers were treated with dressings and compression.

The research showing that over half of these patients actually had reflux in the N2 truncal veins was a major step forward for patients suffering from venous leg ulcers. As we are able to treat reflux in the N2 truncal veins with varicose vein type operations, it meant that we were able to cure at least half of venous leg ulcers by surgically treating the incompetent refluxing superficial veins. Further research has now shown us that venous leg ulcers can come from reflux in the N2 truncal veins, stasis in the N3 superficial veins, reflux in the pelvic veins and reflux in incompetent perforating veins. All of these can be treated under local anaesthetic with modern techniques and research we have published from The Whiteley Clinic has shown that we can cure 85% of venous leg ulcers in patients who can walk, ensuring that most of them never need dressings or compression again.

Randomised controlled trials called the ESCHAR and the EVRA trials have confirmed that in patients with venous leg ulcers, if doctors treat the underlying venous reflux (i.e. the hidden varicose veins) the leg ulcers heal quicker than those treated with compression, and have significantly less chance of ever coming back again.

What is amazing is that despite all of this research, most patients with venous leg ulcers are still only being offered dressings and compression. Hopefully as more patients get to hear about the advances in venous surgery, and hear about patients who have been cured from their venous ulcers with endovenous surgery, we will see increasing numbers of patients being assessed for curative endovenous surgery and reduced numbers been consigned to long-term compression bandaging and dressings.

Although I have used venous leg ulcers as one of the more extreme examples of what hidden varicose veins can cause, it is important that you understand that essentially varicose veins and hidden varicose veins are the same condition. Both are venous reflux due to failed valves in the "superficial" veins of the legs which, as we have discussed before, actually includes any combination of the N2 truncal veins, N3 superficial veins, pelvic veins and perforating veins.

Everyone with venous reflux has blood refluxing abnormally either passively or actively the wrong way through some of their veins in their legs. With time, the reflux increases as the veins dilate, and the clinical condition deteriorates.

When blood refluxes down any of these veins, it can do one of two main things. It can either continue to reflux in the veins deeper under the skin, causing inflammation and damage that will become apparent with time, or it can be diverted into veins nearer the surface that then bulge with the increased flow refluxing back down the veins. These dilating veins near the surface are the varicose veins.

However, if you understand this process, you will see that the development of the varicose veins is secondary to the underlying venous reflux and the bulging varicose veins are not the main problem. Indeed, the varicose veins act as "shock absorbers" stopping the refluxing blood from refluxing straight down to the ankle and causing inflammation. Therefore, the more blood that is refluxing in the leg veins that gets diverted into the bulging varicose veins, the less falls straight down the leg veins to cause inflammation at the ankle.

Thus, the bulging varicose veins seen on the surface are actually protecting the leg, by reducing the volume of refluxing blood getting to the ankle, and therefore reducing the amount of inflammation. Getting rid of varicose veins without getting rid of the underlying reflux worsens the problem.

I always find it quite amusing that patients hate varicose veins and want them removed so that their legs look better, when in fact the varicose veins that they hate are actually working in their favour to reduce the rate of deterioration of their venous disease! This is why one of the chapters in my "understanding venous reflux" book is called "Varicose veins - the good guys!".

Therefore, if you see varicose veins on your legs you should be thankful, because at least you know what is going on in your leg. In addition, you should not be complaining about the varicose veins, but you should be thinking of them as an indication that you have a more severe problem underneath that needs addressing. Fortunately, by addressing that, your varicose veins will also go as they will not be needed any more once the underlying reflux has been cured.

Now that we have explained that varicose veins and hidden varicose veins are virtually the same condition, only different by what is seen on the surface, we can think about what happens if they are left untreated.

Research that I performed in the 1990s and that got into the national newspapers, although unfortunately I did not publish it in medical journals, showed that a sample of schoolgirls that we tested showed 1 in 20 already had venous reflux (hidden varicose veins) at age 9, rising to 1 in 9 at age 18. None in the study had any symptoms and very few had started to show any varicose veins or thread veins on the surface.

However, we know that with time, the conditions deteriorate causing problems we have outlined before.

The deterioration of venous reflux disease (varicose veins or hidden varicose veins) usually follows the course:

- cosmetic varicose veins without any symptoms

and then in all of the following, visible varicose veins may or may not be present:

- thread veins (spider veins or telangiectasia) of the legs particularly around the inner ankle bone

- symptoms in the legs - not usually pain but more often aching, throbbing, heaviness or tiredness of the legs that is improved on lying down

- swelling of the ankle or ankles

- venous eczema - red itchy patches on the lower legs, and sometimes in the upper legs

- a hardness of the lower leg under the calf, often causing shiny skin (called lipodermatosclerosis or LDS) which can give the leg a "champagne bottle" appearance

- red or brown skin stains (haemosiderin deposition) of the lower legs particularly on the inner aspect above the ankle

- a venous leg ulcer that appears as an open sore of the lower leg

This is the basis of a classification system that venous experts use called the "CEAP" classification. However, it is not perfect because there are also other complications from having long-term varicose veins or hidden varicose veins that include:

- bleeding from a varicose vein

- superficial venous thrombosis ("phlebitis")

- deep-vein thrombosis (DVT)

It is a shame that for so many decades doctors and nurses have tried to put patients off having treatment for varicose veins, in the mistaken belief that they are "only cosmetic", do not cause serious problems if left alone and only come back again in the future if treated.

All of these are incorrect, and every patient with symptoms or signs and varicose veins or hidden varicose veins should now be investigated using the latest colour flow duplex ultrasound scanning and treated with a combination of the latest endovenous treatments, to make sure that all of the different sources of reflux are ablated. This is the basis of The Whiteley Protocol®.

All of the reflux in any of these veins can be successfully treated if identified. Currently, although there are two main different approaches to treating veins, the majority of doctors in the northern hemisphere follow what is called an "ablative" approach.

To understand venous ablation, we have to understand that if a vein is refluxing, we know we cannot make it work properly again. We cannot repair the valves and therefore it will always allow venous reflux. Hence the only way we can treat such veins is by permanently ablating them.

In the past, doctors tried to do this by cutting through the skin, finding the vein, and then tying the vein with a surgical ligation. Alternatively, for long truncal veins, the veins were stripped out of the body. Unfortunately, research has shown that this does not work. The surgical ligations slowly break or dissolve, and research that I published in 2007 and again in 2014 shows that any vein that is stripped away has a high chance of growing back again. When it grows back, there are no valves in the new vein and so it is instantly a refluxing vein once again.

In 1999 I introduced the new endovenous surgery into the UK where we use heat to shrivel the vein away and kill it permanently. Our 15-year results published in a peer-reviewed journal shows that once a vein is successfully treated this way, it is permanently closed.

However, this does depend upon the doctor using the correct device that is optimal for the vein being treated and using the right power and pullback combination to completely kill the vein wall. Failure to do this will result in a damaged vein that is not dead, full of thrombus. As the body eats the thrombus away by inflammation, it will slowly repair the vein and over time the vein will re-open and reflux once again.

It is beyond the scope of this book to be exhaustive about all of the different techniques that can be used to ablate refluxing veins, so I will go through some of the techniques that are available to treat the different veins involved in venous reflux.

The N2 truncal veins are the veins that used to be tied at the junction with the N1 veins (the "high tie") whilst the majority of the vein was then stripped away (the "stripping"). As we have seen, this does not work in the majority of patients in the long term and no true venous specialist would offer this to their patients anymore. Indeed, international guidelines from the USA, Europe and UK all agree that it is the least recommended technique to treat varicose veins now.

Nowadays, the optimal treatment for N2 veins is what is called "endovenous thermal ablation". This means putting a device up inside the vein under ultrasound control, local anaesthetic around the vein and then using heat to shrivel the vein away and kill all of the cells. Provided the right technique, power and pullback is used, this should be a permanent cure. The commonest techniques for this are radiofrequency or endovenous laser. More recently steam has been used and in the last couple of years, endovenous microwave has been introduced although this has not fully taken off yet.

There are some other techniques for the N2 truncal veins that do not use heat such as injecting medical superglue (medically called cyanoacrylate glue) into the vein that permanently sticks it together, mechanochemical ablation (MOCA) that uses a combination of trauma to disrupt the inside of the vein and sclerotherapy to kill the cells of the vein wall, or foam sclerotherapy. The medical glue and MOCA have shown some success in some research papers but have not shown enough advantage to become widely adopted by most vein specialists. Foam sclerotherapy has been shown to be much less effective in the treatment of N2 truncal veins than endovenous thermal ablation and so is not used to treat these veins by most vein specialists.

The latest way of treating incompetent N2 veins is a revolutionary and completely non-invasive technique called High Intensity Focused Ultrasound (HIFU) or "Echotherapy" using the Sonovein machine. The Sonovein machine is put on the leg and because it uses ultrasound, gel is put on the skin. However, nothing from the machine physically penetrates the skin. The ultrasound can image the incompetent vein that needs treatment. This is then used to aim a beam of very high intensity ultrasound that is focused just at the vein itself.

The vein is squashed flat with a bit of external pressure and the HIFU fired. This pulse heats the section of vein, completely destroying it and permanently ablating it, just the same as any of the endovenous thermal ablation techniques. The machine is then moved down the leg a few millimetres and the process repeated. If the patient finds it uncomfortable, a very small injection of local anaesthetic can be given around the vein at the point of discomfort. However, this is a tiny injection and is the only part of the procedure that is invasive at all.

Currently this is so new that at the time of writing this book, there are only six machines working in the world. The first research cases were treated in Vienna by Dr Alfred Obermayer, and then the first actual patients treated with this new technique were by myself in the UK in May 2019. A modification of the technique, Sonovein S, was introduced into our clinic in October 2020. This uses a different frequency of ultrasound and has improved the treatment times considerably. It has also reduced patient discomfort, meaning we use a lot less local anaesthetic. In some patients, we don't need local anaesthetic at all.

N3 superficial veins are generally treated by either removing the vein by hooking it out ("phlebectomy") or destroying it using foam sclerotherapy. Generally, if the vein wall is thick or the vein large, phlebectomy is used to physically remove it through a tiny hole, usually only about 2 mm long. If the vein is smaller, and thin walled, then foam sclerotherapy can be injected into it to destroy it.

However, to get good results from foam sclerotherapy you need to wear compression for some time after the injection, with studies suggesting 2-3 weeks being optimal. Foam sclerotherapy in large veins tends to cause permanent brown stains and so this is why phlebectomy is still used in those veins. Neither technique is perfect and often we will use a combination of both to get the best results for patients. Without doubt, a new technique is needed to treat these superficial N3 veins.

Incompetent perforating veins are best treated using a technique that was invented by myself and Judy Holdstock in 2001 called TRLOP (TRansLuminal Occlusion of Perforators). This was "re-invented" in America in 2007 and re-named PAPS (perforator ablation procedure) although it is clearly exactly the same technique just re-named.

An ultrasound is used to guide a needle into the incompetent perforating vein. A device is then placed into the vein such as a radiofrequency or laser, although other people have used medical glue. If one of the heating methods is used, local anaesthetic is then injected around the vein. The vein is then ablated. Hence, an incompetent perforator vein can now be treated under ultrasound control and under local anaesthetic, leaving no visible scar.

One of the interesting developments of incompetent perforating vein treatments is that HIFU is also very effective for treating these veins. As this is non-invasive and quick with the new Sonovein S machine, this may become a standard treatment for these veins in the future.

Incompetent pelvic veins are best treated by what is called "coil embolisation". Under local anaesthetic, a catheter is passed from a single needle hole in the right side of the neck, down through the venous system and into the pelvic veins. Platinum coils are then pushed into the pelvic varicose veins, completely blocking them. Although platinum coils are expensive, they are the least likely metal to cause any allergic response. As they are going to stay inside permanently, this is essential. Some patients ask if absorbable coils can be used but this is not logical. It is a bit like asking for an absorbable hip replacement! As soon as the coils absorb, new ones would have to be put in place.

You may wonder why we use coils rather than laser, as laser is so effective in leg veins. The problem with endovenous laser or any other heat method is that if you heat the veins in the pelvis, you can damage other surrounding structures such as the bowel, nerves, bladder or other pelvic structures. This does not happen in the legs as we can inject local anaesthetic around the outside of the leg vein during the treatment. However, we cannot do this in the pelvic veins.

There are other techniques that are becoming available and many people are using combinations of lasers and foam sclerotherapy, or other sorts of material that are implanted in the body. However, so far none of them have undergone rigorous testing. The above techniques are the most well-known used by venous specialists who are involved in research and development, and who audit their results. Venous surgery is a fast-moving subject, and so new techniques may well become available and standard in the near future.

Post thrombotic syndrome (PTS) and deep vein reflux

Fortunately, post thrombotic syndrome and deep vein reflux (N1 veins) is not terribly common. We have discussed this previously but to recap, it is almost always found in patients who have had either a very extensive deep vein thrombosis that was not treated quickly and aggressively, or who have had recurrent deep vein thromboses in the past.

Whichever reason, it is the long-term inflammation that the thrombus causes in the vein wall that ends up causing scarring of the vein, that causes the problem.

As we discussed previously, initially it was thought that the scarring caused the valves in the deep veins to fail, resulting in deep vein reflux.

However, more recent work over the last one or two decades has shown that the symptoms and signs of PTS are more often due to obstruction from scar tissue, either partially or completely blocking the deep veins in the leg (N1) or pelvic veins, with the deep-vein reflux being only a side issue.

Therefore, traditionally doctors (even consultants specialising in "vascular surgery") have regarded deep vein problems as incurable, and only ever recommended long-term compression.

However, increasing number of specialists are now diagnosing the venous obstruction in patients with PTS, and are opening these obstructions by dilating them with balloons under x-ray control, and then keeping them open with metal network tubes called stents. This area is still relatively new, but we have seen some amazing successes in patients who have had huge swollen legs with leg ulcers for years and who were unable to walk more than 20 or 30 metres because of pain on walking. Such patients often get back to an almost normal lifestyle if they are suitable for stenting. What is surprising is that the deep vein reflux is still present but turns out to be virtually irrelevant once the obstruction has been removed.

Superficial venous thrombosis ("phlebitis")

I am astounded that we have not seen more complaints, and even legal actions, over the poor management that most patients seem to get when they have superficial venous thrombosis or "phlebitis".

As we have already discussed previously, superficial venous thrombosis which is commonly called "phlebitis" presents as a red, hot, tender, lump on the leg, commonly in a place where a varicose vein has been seen previously. As we have said before, the presentation can vary a little depending on the extent of the thrombus or depth of the vein affected.

Again, to reiterate what we have said before, it is a blood clot (thrombosis) in the affected vein causing inflammation and is not anything to do with infection.

Treatment with antibiotics is wrong.

Treatment depends on how far the clot has extended. Guidelines published in the USA and UK in 2012 are very clear on this matter.

If the clot is in, or extends into, one of the N2 truncal veins, and is within 5 cm of the junction with the N1 deep veins, then there is a 1% chance that the clot will embolise to the lungs - a pulmonary embolism. This is a serious condition that can be life threatening. As such, the recommendations are very clear.

If the superficial venous thrombosis is only in the N3 veins, or is in the N2 truncal veins but over 5-7 cm away from the junction with the deep N1 veins, then the patient should be treated with non-steroidal anti-inflammatory drugs if they are able to take them (such as aspirin or ibuprofen) which will act as both a painkiller and anti-inflammatory. They will also be prescribed compression stockings. The compression stockings will help with the discomfort and also help increase the speed of blood flow in the superficial and deep veins, reducing the risk of clot propagation.

However, if the superficial venous thrombosis is in an N2 truncal vein and does extend within 5 cm or closer to the junction with an N1 deep vein, then the patient should have full anticoagulation to reduce the risk of pulmonary embolism. Compression stockings may also be given for comfort, but the anticoagulation is the most important factor.

In both cases, once the superficial venous thrombosis has resolved, the patient should be scanned formally and any underlying varicose veins or hidden varicose veins should be treated to prevent the problem occurring again.

As you will see from the above description, very few patients who present with "phlebitis" get the right treatment. Many still get antibiotics. Many will get non-steroidal anti-inflammatory medication and compression stockings but will not be sent for a colour flow duplex ultrasound scan and so will never know if they should have been anticoagulated. Hence a proportion of patients presenting to doctors with "phlebitis" will suffer from a pulmonary embolism which could have been avoided.

It is amazing to me that although the guidelines have been published for over eight years now, most doctors and nurses seem unaware of this change in understanding and treatment. As with many areas of medicine, it will only be by complaints and suing that most doctors and nurses will eventually change their practice.

Deep vein thrombosis (DVT)

We have looked at this quite extensively before and so I will not reiterate too much in this chapter, but only add a few new items that I have not mentioned previously.

To recap on previous chapters, deep-vein thrombosis is the formation of a clot in the deep veins (N1) of the legs, or pelvic veins. The thrombus can be partial or complete. It can extend if left untreated and can either break off completely or part of it break off, flying up through the venous system to the right side of the heart and then onto the lungs causing a pulmonary embolism.

Local symptoms in the leg are caused by local inflammation from the clot irritating the vein wall, and obstruction of the flow usually causing an aching and swelling downstream from where the clot is.

The lower the deep vein thrombosis in the leg, the smaller the clot and the less significant the swelling, symptoms and potential danger. The higher the deep vein thrombosis in the leg or pelvis, the larger the clot and the more significant the swelling, symptoms and potential danger.

Diagnosis is ideally by colour flow venous duplex ultrasound scan. In specialist centres this is done immediately so that appropriate treatment can be started.

To save money and to streamline services, many hospitals and emergency departments now perform a blood test called a D-dimer test. This test looks for the products of blood clotting in the veins. If it is negative, a deep vein thrombosis is unlikely. If positive, a deep vein thrombosis is possible or likely and so anticoagulation treatment is started, usually as an injection of heparin once a day, but sometimes nowadays an oral tablet that causes anticoagulation.

As we discussed before, this treatment does not affect the deep vein thrombosis itself but stops any propagation of new clot forming on the old. This also allows time for the body to start breaking down the clot itself by its own thrombolysis (clot splitting) system.

Patients with a positive D-dimer are usually started on anti-coagulant treatment and are then invited back for a colour flow venous duplex ultrasound scan on the next available list.

Most research accepts that deep vein thromboses are best treated by anticoagulation. However, because of the risks of post-thrombotic syndrome, particularly in patients with large deep vein thromboses in the thigh veins or pelvic veins, there are trials looking at different ways of removing the clot using catheters to either physically remove it or use drugs to break down the clot. Currently there is no clear answer as to which technique is better, and so the standard way is still anticoagulation. However, this may change if clot removal is perfected.

We have now covered most of the underlying causes looking at both venous reflux under the heading of varicose veins and hidden varicose veins, and clots under superficial venous thrombosis and deep vein thrombosis. As you'll see, there is a lot of crossover between different venous conditions and causes, with venous leg ulcers, phlebitis and other related conditions figuring to an extent in both areas. This is because there is a crossover between any underlying causes for venous disease and the complications that can occur.

However, if you have read through all of the book so far, hopefully you will have a fairly clear idea of the venous system, how it works normally, how it can go wrong in terms of reflux, stasis, obstruction and how that can cause inflammation or clotting.

Although everything written so far is appropriate to anyone with venous disease in normal life, regardless of lockdown or isolation, in the next short chapter I'm going to briefly discuss Covid-19 and blood clots.

After that, I am going to bring this book to a close with a summary and an attempt to pull all the strands I have explored together. I will try and give an overall idea of how quickly you should seek help if you think you have any of the venous problems we have discussed.

Chapter 8

Covid-19 and venous thrombosis

So far, everything in this book relates to venous disease that we see every day in clinical practice. I have written this book as some of these conditions can be exacerbated in a lockdown or isolation. As many people are very scared of seeking medical advice during these periods, I hope it will help people assess whether they need urgent care or will be safe to postpone seeking advice.

However, there is a direct effect of the Covid-19 infection on venous thrombosis which is different from normal venous disease.

When the Covid pandemic started in the Western world in early 2020, it was initially thought to be a virus that affected the respiratory system, much the same as an influenza type virus.

However, reports from Italy initially, and then from the United States showed that in very sick patients, blood clots were appearing far more frequently in patients sick with Covid-19 than would be expected in people who were just as sick, but with other conditions such as flu.

These blood clots were mainly thromboses in the venous system, although some were found in the arteries. In some of the early research papers published on the subject, most of the thromboses were found in the veins in the lungs, preventing oxygen getting into the bloodstream. This showed why doctors had not been successful in ventilating such patients. When patients with respiratory illnesses have low blood oxygen, it is usual for doctors to put a tube into the lungs called "intubation" and then ventilate the patient, forcing oxygen into the lungs with a ventilator.

However, although this might work when there is a problem like infection or inflammation in the lung tissue, it doesn't work if the veins have all thrombosed and blood is not circulating in the lungs at all. Any oxygen forced into the lungs cannot get into the blood, if all of the veins in the lungs are blocked with thrombus.

Whenever doctors see clot in the pulmonary veins in the lungs, they always think that it comes from deep vein thrombosis as we have discussed previously in this book. However, it quickly became apparent that the pulmonary thrombosis in the veins in the lungs in patients suffering from Covid-19 were widespread throughout the lungs, and most patients did not have any corresponding deep vein thromboses. Therefore, it soon became apparent that in patients who are very sick with Covid-19, a proportion of these patients are developing thromboses directly in the veins in the lungs as a result of the infection.

A webinar that I was involved in, in early summer 2020, discussed this in great detail. One of the speakers, Joseph Caprini, who is one of the most famous doctors in understanding venous thrombosis in the world, and the host of the webinar from South America, explained that in very sick patients they were performing a D-dimer blood test on admission, to see if there was any evidence of generalised venous thrombosis in their sickest patients. Any of the sick patients suspected of having Covid-19, with a positive D-dimer, was then anticoagulated to keep the pulmonary circulation flowing to enable oxygen to continue to flow into the bloodstream.

As with many medical tests, a raised D-dimer is not specific for venous thrombosis and can be elevated for other reasons including inflammation.

However, when dealing with people who have suspected Covid-19, and who are very unwell, a raised D-dimer was certainly strong evidence that anticoagulation may well help keep them alive.

As 2020 has gone on, more papers have been written on the link between Covid-19 and venous thrombosis.

People who have mild illness seem to have either very low or non-existent risk of venous thrombosis. We have reported a case of a man who appears to have thrombosed a testicular vein, and there are one or two other cases that are coming to light in patients infected with Covid-19 but mild enough symptoms to be treated at home.

Patients with Covid-19 who are ill enough to need hospital admission have a higher rate of venous thrombosis, and those that need intensive care have a very significant risk of severe venous thrombosis.

In these very sick patients, the majority of the venous thromboses are in the pulmonary veins in the lung, with a small proportion of cases having deep vein thrombosis in the legs. There are other sites of thrombosis that have been reported. Patients with arterial disease have also been reported as having severe arterial thrombosis, if very sick with Covid-19.

However, as far as this book is concerned, if you are at home either during a lockdown or isolating, and either do not have Covid-19 or find that you are positive but have very mild symptoms, then the risks of a venous thrombosis due to the Covid-19 appear to be very small or even non-existent.

Therefore, although you should take all of the lessons in this book to heart regarding veins and venous disease and any symptoms you may notice either at this time or in the future, there is little specific to Covid-19 infection unless you are very unwell and admitted to hospital.

Chapter 9

Keeping your veins healthy and when to look for help

Much of venous disease is a chronic deterioration of the venous system, in those who are susceptible. This is because the commonest venous problems stem from the valves failing in the leg veins, causing venous reflux. As we have seen, this can cause dilated veins (varicose veins) but this only happens in about half the patients with venous reflux. The others have the hidden version of varicose veins.

In all patients with venous reflux, if the reflux is allowed to continue (i.e. patients do not get treated), then the medical condition of the leg can worsen due to inflammation around the ankles and lower legs, and acute episodes can happen causing bleeding or clots.

As we have noted, there are other less common causes of venous disease as well, including venous stasis and obstruction of the venous system flowing out of the legs.

Although you may have bought this book because of a lockdown or isolation, almost all of the information in it is actually relevant to everybody all of the time. However, when people change lifestyles and are at home more often than usual, and may have other changes such as changing diet and exercise, then rapid changes can occur in those people with venous disease, even if they weren't aware that they had a problem with their veins previously.

Of course, there are other conditions that affect the legs that might be mistaken for venous disease. In early summer 2020 I saw an emergency case of a 34 year old lady who had been in lockdown in her flat. She had been trying to exercise as best as she could without going out. At that stage the UK government was telling people not to go out for more than one hour at a time. One of the exercises that she did was to lie on her back, raise her legs in the air and then cycle her legs. She found that when she did this, one of her legs went numb. Her aunt recommended she come to see me as an emergency as she thought it might be something to do with her veins. However, I found that she had a completely blocked artery in her thigh. She was lucky not to have lost her leg already and I had her admitted urgently to open up the artery or perform bypass as needed.

Another patient who had severe varicose veins and had been seeing a doctor elsewhere for regular foam sclerotherapy treatment (which wasn't having any effect), started developing a patch of rough skin on the front of her leg. Because all of the medical consultations that she could arrange with her family doctor were online, she had been told that this was probably eczema. When she came to see me, it was clear that this was a basal cell carcinoma of the skin and she was referred urgently for removal of this skin cancer. This is one of the skin cancers that can be associated, albeit rarely, with chronic inflammation secondary to varicose veins and more usually venous leg ulcers.

I am sure that any other doctor who sees many vein patients will have their own stories and so it must be remembered that not all leg problems are necessarily due to veins or are solely venous conditions. However, venous disease is very common in the population, and is often underestimated as a cause of severe leg problems.

Throughout this book I have hopefully explained how to keep your veins healthy, and more importantly I hope I have explained how veins work normally and what can go wrong with them. If you understand the underlying principles, then you will be able to understand why the things that are helpful work, and you will be able to see through bad advice or sales pitches.

For the final part of this book, I will now try to give an indication as to what conditions need treatment, and more importantly with what urgency. If you are reading this outside of a lockdown or isolation, then it will help you know if you should seek medical help and what help you should ask for.

If you are reading this during a lockdown or isolation, I will indicate which ones constitute a medical emergency or urgent case and should cause you to seek urgent medical care despite any lockdown or isolation regulations.

Although in Chapter 7 we went through the underlying causes, these are not particularly useful to you unless you know what sort of underlying venous disease you might have. Therefore, I am going to base my advice on the assessment you will make yourself of your legs by following the symptoms and signs as we discussed in Chapter 2:

Aching, heavy or tired legs (with or without varicose veins)

Although these are fairly good symptoms of varicose veins or hidden varicose veins, and are indications for colour flow duplex ultrasonography and treatment if reflux is found according to international guidelines, these symptoms do not constitute an urgent problem by themselves. Therefore, if these are the only symptoms you have:

- **Outside of a lockdown or isolation** - you should book a consultation and scan at a specialist vein clinic as a routine case.

- **During lockdown or isolation** - you do not need to seek urgent medical help and should wait until after lockdown or isolation finishes, unless your lockdown rules allow for medical consultations and treatments. Continue to exercise, elevate your legs and consider compression stockings along with the other home help advice in this book. However, you should book a consultation and scan at a specialist vein clinic for when the lockdown or your isolation is finished.

Thread veins/spider veins on leg or ankle

Most people with thread veins or spider veins on their legs or ankles have underlying venous reflux, either varicose veins or hidden varicose veins. If there are no other symptoms or signs at all, this is a purely cosmetic problem and does not fulfil the medical criteria for medical treatment. As such, they do not constitute an urgent medical problem.

Please note that if you do have other symptoms or signs, please look up the section on the relevant symptoms or signs. This advice is for those with thread veins/ spider veins only.

Although not medically necessary, you can have your veins treated for cosmetic reasons. To get the optimal treatment for your veins, you will need to have a colour flow duplex ultrasound scan to see if you are one of the majority of people who have underlying venous reflux (hidden varicose veins) and if you are, you should have the venous reflux treated before starting any treatment for the thread veins. If you do not have underlying venous reflux, you can start on thread vein treatments immediately. The most effective way of treating leg thread veins is microsclerotherapy.

- **Outside of a lockdown or isolation** - there is no medical indication for any treatment. If you want treatment for cosmetic purposes, you should book a consultation and colour flow venous duplex ultrasound scan to look for underlying venous reflux. The underlying venous reflux should be treated first, followed by the leg thread veins by microsclerotherapy.

- **During lockdown or isolation** - there is no medical indication for needing help during a lockdown or isolation. See above for what to do outside of a lockdown or isolation.

Profuse green veins over the legs that may be associated with thread veins

If this is the only sign that you have, with no other symptoms, then the advice is the same as for thread veins and spider veins. There is no medical reason for investigation and treatment but if you want a cosmetic improvement, you can attend a specialist vein clinic which will scan you looking for underlying reflux and then formulate a plan of treatment appropriate for you.

- **Outside of a lockdown or isolation** - there is no medical indication for any treatment. If you want treatment for cosmetic purposes, you should book a consultation and colour flow venous duplex ultrasound scan to look for underlying venous reflux. The underlying venous reflux should be treated first, followed by planned treatment for the other veins as appropriate.

- **During lockdown or isolation** - there is no medical indication for needing help during a lockdown or isolation. See above for what to do outside of a lockdown or isolation.

Varicose veins of the legs with no symptoms

Bulging veins of the legs that are seen on standing, which are visible varicose veins, are not an indication for treatment by themselves. Indeed, if you have no symptoms at all, but just do not like the bulging varicose veins, then there is no medical necessity for you to have any treatment at all.

Of course as you will have seen from the previous chapters, these bulging veins are almost always due to underlying venous reflux and with time, you will develop symptoms and signs that will lead to a medical requirement for treatment.

However, the current research and guidelines states that if you do not have any symptoms or signs apart from bulging varicose veins, then there is no medical need for treatment. If you want these veins treated for cosmetic reasons, then you can do so but outside of a lockdown or isolation.

- **Outside of a lockdown or isolation** - there is no medical indication for any treatment. If you want treatment for cosmetic purposes, you should book a consultation and colour flow venous duplex ultrasound scan at a specialist vein clinic to identify what pattern of disease you have. The doctor should then be able to recommend the appropriate treatment for your specific pattern of reflux.

- **During lockdown or isolation** - there is no medical indication for needing help during a lockdown or isolation. See above for what to do outside of a lockdown or isolation.

Varicose veins of the vulva, vagina, scrotum, buttocks

If you notice these veins appear, but there are no other symptoms or signs, they will need investigation and possible treatment but not as an urgent case. If any of them are painful, or develop hard, tender, swollen lumps, then this should be regarded as a thrombosis and the advice should be taken under superficial venous thrombosis or "phlebitis" rather than this section.

Therefore, this section is for varicose veins that have appeared in these areas **that are not causing any symptoms or other signs at all**.

- **Outside of a lockdown or isolation** - you should book to see a vein specialist in a vein centre that specialises in pelvic veins and you will need to undergo investigations. Optimally these are transvaginal or transabdominal colour flow duplex ultrasound scans using the Holdstock-Harrison and Holdstock-White protocols, often after bowel preparation so the veins can be seen clearly. Some doctors use CT, MRI or venography although these are not as useful. However, in some patients they can be used to get additional information to help with the diagnosis. Treatment will depend on the results.

- **During lockdown or isolation** - there is no medical indication for needing help during a lockdown or isolation, unless your lockdown rules allow for medical consultations and treatments. See above for what to do outside of a lockdown or isolation.

Haemorrhoids (piles)

As we discussed in Chapter 2, haemorrhoids are traditionally treated by bowel surgeons because of where they appear. However, some of our research has suggested that haemorrhoids might be more linked with pelvic varicose veins than bowel problems, and so venous surgeons and phlebologists are becoming more interested in this area.

As far as this book is concerned at this time, just having the appearance of haemorrhoids (piles) as bulging veins from the anus is not an urgent problem.

However, if they thrombose (suddenly go very hard and painful) or bleed profusely, then these become medical emergencies and you should seek emergency help even in a lockdown or during isolation.

- **Outside of a lockdown or isolation** – if you have noticed haemorrhoids you should seek medical advice. At your appointment, the doctor will check that there is no other problem associated with the haemorrhoids, and in the most modern clinics, will offer you local anaesthetic treatment with radiofrequency ablation or banding.

- **During lockdown or isolation** – you should only seek urgent medical help if the haemorrhoids become very painful and go hard, or if they start to bleed significantly. In these cases, contact your family doctor or go to the emergency room. For haemorrhoids that are not painful and have not changed for a while, see above for what to do outside of a lockdown or isolation.

Varicose veins of the abdomen or flank

Varicose veins over the lower abdomen, around the umbilicus (belly-button) or up the flanks are usually a sign of a blocked vein inside the pelvis or abdomen. They can also be a sign of liver disease.

If these veins have been there for a long time and there has been no sudden change, they should certainly be investigated but probably can wait for a few weeks if you are in the middle of a lockdown or isolation, unless your lockdown rules allow for medical consultations and treatments. However, if the veins have suddenly appeared, or have suddenly worsened, or you have any other symptoms or signs, you should contact a medical professional to discuss these and have them assessed urgently.

- **Outside of a lockdown or isolation** - these sorts of veins need to be investigated to find out what is going on to cause them. You should contact your family doctor or a venous specialist to arrange a consultation and appropriate investigations that will probably start off with a colour flow duplex ultrasound scan. This should be done with the matter of some urgency unless you have had the veins for a long time and they have not changed, in which case it can be done in a more relaxed manner.

- **During lockdown or isolation** - if these veins have appeared suddenly, or there are any other signs or symptoms associated with them, you should get medical advice urgently. You should contact your family doctor or a venous specialist clinic and arrange an urgent consultation and colour flow duplex ultrasound scan. If however the veins have been there for some time and have not changed, and there are no other signs or symptoms, you should be able to wait till after lockdown or isolation to attend a consultation, unless your lockdown rules allow you to attend medical appointments. If unsure, contact a doctor for advice.

Varicose veins of the chest, arms, hands, breasts or face

These sorts of veins usually develop slowly and without any other sorts of symptoms. They are generally only a cosmetic problem and should be seen by vein specialists who specialise in cosmetic vein work. Therefore, for any of these sorts of veins that have been there for some time, are not tender, not particularly swollen and do not have any associated inflammation or swelling, then there is no medical indication for any treatment. However, they can be treated for cosmetic reasons by a specialist who does cosmetic venous work.

- **Outside of a lockdown or isolation** - there is no medical indication for any treatment. If you want treatment for cosmetic purposes, you should book a consultation with a venous specialist who specialises in venous cosmetic work.

- **During lockdown or isolation** - there is no medical indication for needing help during a lockdown or isolation. See above for what to do outside of a lockdown or isolation.

Sudden swollen and tender veins appearing over shoulder, chest and upper arm

The major exception to the advice given above for arm veins is if veins suddenly appear over the shoulder or upper arm or chest and are tender, or there is swelling of the arm. If this happens, it is often a sign that there has been a deep vein thrombosis in the arm vein. In this sort of situation, you will need to have very urgent treatment either through the emergency department or through an urgent appointment with a vein clinic, if they take urgent cases. Indeed this should be treated the same as a deep vein thrombosis of the leg:

- **Outside of a lockdown or isolation** - a sudden swelling of veins over the shoulder, chest and upper arm, with or without swelling of the arm suggests a deep vein thrombosis of the arm vein. You should consult the emergency services for urgent assessment or go to an emergency appointment at a vein clinic if they provide emergency appointments.

- **During lockdown or isolation** - a sudden swelling of veins over the shoulder, chest and upper arm, with or without swelling of the arm suggests a deep vein thrombosis of the arm vein. You should consult the emergency services for urgent assessment or go to an emergency appointment at a vein clinic if they provide emergency appointments.

Swelling of part or all of one lower limb

Sudden swelling of one leg should be a cause of great concern. In particular, if there is any discomfort, or pain in the muscle during active or passive movement, then these are even more worrying signs.

Within the text of this book we have discussed that the position and size of any deep vein thrombosis can vary the position and extent of any swelling, and also any discomfort that is felt. In addition, there are other conditions such as a ruptured Bakers cyst (an out-pouching of the knee joint into the area behind the knee that can rupture irritating the calf muscle) that can cause pain and swelling in the leg.

However, for safety reasons, any sudden and unexpected swelling of one leg should be considered to be a deep vein thrombosis until proven not to be. The presence of any discomfort or pain is also worrying, but should not stop you seeking medical advice.

Of course, if you have banged your leg or have any other known reason for the swelling, then you might want to discuss this with your doctor. However, unless you are certain you know the reason for the swelling, then one must assume it is a deep vein thrombosis until proven otherwise.

- **Outside of a lockdown or isolation** - sudden swelling of one leg should be considered to be a possible deep vein thrombosis. You should attend the emergency room or have an urgent appointment at a specialist vein clinic if they give emergency appointments for deep vein thrombosis.

- **During lockdown or isolation** - as this is a medical emergency, the same advice is applicable even during a lockdown or during isolation. You should attend the emergency room or have an urgent appointment at a specialist vein clinic if they give emergency appointments for deep vein thrombosis.

Eczema of the lower leg just above the ankle (with or without varicose veins being visible)

Eczema of the lower leg just above the ankle, or indeed eczema anywhere on the leg, must be considered to be venous eczema until proven otherwise. If you have eczema elsewhere on the body, then venous eczema is less likely. If however you do not have eczema anywhere else, and just on one or both legs, venous eczema is more likely.

Venous eczema is caused by the inflammation of venous reflux or venous stasis. It is an indication for medical treatment of venous reflux (varicose veins or hidden varicose veins). However, although it is a medical problem, it is not an urgent medical condition that would need to break a lockdown or isolation, unless your lockdown rules allow for medical consultations and treatments.

- **Outside of a lockdown or isolation** - you should book a consultation and colour flow venous duplex ultrasound scan with a venous specialist to diagnose your venous disease and to plan appropriate treatment.

- **During lockdown or isolation** - there is no indication for urgent medical assessment during a lockdown or isolation, unless your lockdown rules allow for medical consultations and treatments. Venous eczema is a medical condition and so if medical appointments are allowed, you should book a consultation and colour flow venous duplex ultrasound scan with a venous specialist to diagnose your venous disease and to plan appropriate treatment. If your rules do not allow you to attend medical appointments, then make the appointment for when you are allowed to travel again.

Red or brown skin changes around the ankle

Red or brown skin changes around the ankles, particularly on the inside of the lower leg below the calf and above the ankle joint, are caused by the inflammation of venous reflux disease or venous stasis. They rarely appear suddenly and have usually been there sometime even if they are slowly worsening.

Although this sort of skin damage constitutes a medical need for investigation and treatment of the venous disease, this is not needed urgently enough to break a lockdown or isolation, unless your lockdown rules allow for medical consultations and treatments.

- **Outside of a lockdown or isolation** - you should book a consultation and colour flow venous duplex ultrasound scan with a venous specialist to diagnose your venous disease and to plan appropriate treatment.

- **During lockdown or isolation** - there is no indication for urgent medical assessment during a lockdown or isolation, unless your lockdown rules allow for medical consultations and treatments. However, as this is a medical condition, if you know when the lockdown is going to finish, or your isolation is going to end, you should book a consultation and colour flow venous duplex ultrasound scan when you are allowed to travel again, with a venous specialist to diagnose your venous disease and to plan appropriate treatment. If your lockdown does allow you to attend medical appointments, then as this is a medical condition, you should book your consultation and scan to prevent further deterioration.

Hard shiny skin just above the ankle

Hard shiny skin above the ankle, that if it is severe enough may cause constriction and make the lower leg look like an inverted "champagne bottle", is called lipodermatosclerosis. It is another sign of inflammation of the tissue around the ankle caused by venous reflux disease or venous stasis.

It is recognised as a sign that indicates the need to be treated for medical reasons. However, it is not an acute problem and does not need you to break a lockdown or isolation, unless your lockdown rules allow for medical consultations and treatments. However, it is a medical problem and as soon as you are able to travel and attend a routine medical appointment, you should do so.

- **Outside of a lockdown or isolation** - you should book a consultation and colour flow venous duplex ultrasound scan with a venous specialist to diagnose your venous disease and to plan appropriate treatment.

- **During lockdown or isolation** - there is no indication for urgent medical assessment during a lockdown or isolation, unless your lockdown rules allow for medical consultations and treatments. However, as this is a medical condition, if you know when the lockdown is going to finish, or your isolation is going to end, you should book a consultation and colour flow venous duplex ultrasound scan when you are allowed to travel again, with a venous specialist to diagnose your venous disease and to plan appropriate treatment. If your lockdown does allow you to attend medical appointments, then as this is a medical condition, you should book your consultation and scan to prevent further deterioration.

Sudden appearance of tender lumps of the legs that may be colourless or red

The sudden appearance of tender lumps on one leg, or very occasionally both legs, is usually the sign of "phlebitis" or superficial venous thrombosis. The usual signs are lumps that are red, hot, tender and swollen locally. As we have discussed previously, these lumps might be too deep to be red, and you might not see the swelling.

As noted previously, if the thrombus encroaches on the deep vein, there is a 1% risk of a clot flying to the lung (pulmonary embolism). Therefore, you should now have an urgent colour flow venous duplex ultrasound scan to see whether you need anticoagulation or not.

Unfortunately, many doctors and nurses are unaware of these guidelines even though they have been published since 2012, and you may need to push to make sure you get the correct investigation and treatment. Because of the risk of pulmonary embolism in patients with "phlebitis" or superficial venous thrombosis, you should attend an emergency room or a specialist venous clinic for an urgent scan and assessment as to whether you need anticoagulation or not. You should also plan to have the underlying venous reflux treated in the long term to stop the problem happening again.

- **Outside of a lockdown or isolation** - the appearance of tender lumps on the legs represents superficial venous thrombosis and you should have an urgent colour flow duplex ultrasound scan to see if you need anticoagulation or not.

- **During lockdown or isolation** - the appearance of tender lumps on the legs represents superficial venous thrombosis and you should have an urgent colour flow duplex ultrasound scan to see if you need anticoagulation or not. Because there is a risk of pulmonary embolism, and you may need anticoagulation, this is an indication to leave your home for medical assessment even during a lockdown or isolation.

An open sore on the lower leg or foot (called an ulcer)

A venous leg ulcer is usually something that occurs slowly over time and is rarely an emergency. Even if it has only just appeared, it usually happens in an area of the leg that has previously shown signs of chronic venous disease such as a red stain, brown stain or a hard patch of skin and hard underlying tissue.

As long as you are able to walk, most venous leg ulcers can now be cured by treating the underlying venous reflux, venous stasis or uncommonly, venous obstruction.

Unless there is any acute change such as infection or swelling of the leg, an open sore or venous ulcer of the leg or foot needs medical investigation and treatment, but not urgently. However, if your lockdown rules allow medical consultations and treatments, you should book an appointment at a specialist vein clinic so that you can get the ulcer healed as quickly as possible.

- **Outside of a lockdown or isolation** - all venous leg ulcers should be investigated in a specialist venous clinic. You should book a consultation and colour flow duplex ultrasound scan so that you can be assessed for curative surgery or informed as to why curative surgery cannot be performed.

- **During lockdown or isolation** - unless there is any sudden change, a venous leg ulcer is not an emergency that needs you to leave your house during lockdown or isolation, unless your lockdown rules allow for medical consultations and treatments.

Most venous leg ulcers can be cured by investigation and endovenous surgery, and so you should book a consultation and colour flow duplex ultrasound scan to be assessed. If you do have any pain, swelling or infection in the ulcer, or if there has been a sudden change in your ulcer, then these are indications for you to seek an urgent opinion and you should be able to attend urgent consultations and assessments during a lockdown or during isolation.

Profuse bleeding of dark blood from a bulging vein on the leg or foot

Bleeding from a varicose vein is definitely a medical emergency!

As veins only have pressure in them when they are below the heart, the first thing to do is to lie down and elevate your leg so the bleeding point is as high as possible above the heart. Direct pressure on the bleeding point can also stop the bleeding.

You should call an ambulance to attend an emergency department immediately or attend a vein clinic urgently if they take emergencies and you can be taken there safely. In the short-term the bleeding needs to be stopped. The underlying cause, usually venous reflux, needs to be identified with a colour flow duplex ultrasound scan and then the veins treated to stop this happening again.

- **Outside of a lockdown or isolation** - you should attend an emergency room or specialist vein clinic if they accept emergency patients for bleeding. You will need a colour flow venous duplex ultrasound scan and acute treatment to stop the bleeding. You will then need planned treatment of the underlying venous reflux to stop this happening again.

- **During lockdown or isolation** - you should attend an emergency room or specialist vein clinic if they accept emergency patients for bleeding. You will need a colour flow venous duplex ultrasound scan and acute treatment to stop the bleeding. You will then need planned treatment of the underlying venous reflux to stop this happening again.

Swelling particularly of the toes on one or both sides

Swelling of the legs that goes right down to the toes on one or both sides is often lymphoedema. It is uncommon for lymphoedema to occur suddenly and so there is usually a longer history of swelling.

If you have certain swelling and have not had the problem before, then please see the section above about certain swelling of the leg or legs. However, if you have swelling of one or both legs and it has been going on for some time, and this goes all the way to the toes, you may well have lymphoedema. This should be investigated and you should have venous reflux excluded as part of this investigation, as both lymphoedema and venous reflux can coexist in the same patient. If both are found, the venous reflux can be treated and, if the lymphodema is still significant, then lymphatic treatments can be started.

Although this is a medical condition, it does not need to be treated urgently during a lockdown or during isolation unless there has been a sudden change such as infection, increased temperature or pain, unless your lockdown rules allow for medical consultations and treatments.

- **Outside of a lockdown or isolation** - you should arrange a consultation and scan with a lymphoedema and venous specialist to ensure that you have your lymphatics and your veins investigated.

- **During lockdown or isolation** - there is no medical reason to have investigation and treatment during a lockdown or isolation, unless your lockdown rules allow for medical consultations and treatments, OR unless there has been a sudden change such as infection, increased temperature or pain.

Swelling of both legs exactly the same on each side

As we discussed in Chapter 2, swelling of both legs makes deep-vein thrombosis less likely, although it is possible.

Therefore, this is one of the areas where you will need to make your own decision, based on the information you have been given in this book.

If your legs were completely normal and suddenly swelled, and particularly if the swelling is quite significant and there is any discomfort, then obviously something acute has happened and you need to have an emergency assessment. You might have deep-vein thrombosis on both sides or there may be some other cause for your bilateral leg swelling. If the change has been sudden, you are definitely a medical emergency and need to contact an urgent or emergency medical team so you can be appropriately investigated and treated.

- **Outside of a lockdown or isolation** - sudden swelling of both legs, particularly if the swelling is significant and there is any discomfort, means you should be seen as an urgent or emergency case in emergency room or specialist vein clinic if they provide an emergency service.

- **During lockdown or isolation** - sudden swelling of both legs, particularly if the swelling is significant and there is any discomfort, means you should be seen as an urgent or emergency case in the emergency room or specialist vein clinic if they provide an emergency service. As this is an urgent or emergency case, you should be seen even during a lockdown or if you are isolating.

If the swelling has been coming on over some time, and is quite mild, and is not associated with any pain or discomfort, then it can probably be investigated as a fairly routine problem.

- **Outside of a lockdown or isolation** - if you have had swelling of both legs for some time, and particularly if it is mild swelling and not associated with any pain or discomfort, then you should be investigated in due course. You should book an appointment with your family doctor or if you are suspicious that it could be venous disease, with a vein specialist for a consultation and probable colour flow duplex ultrasound scan.

- **During lockdown or isolation** - for swelling that has taken some time to develop and is quite mild, there is no reason for this to be investigated during a lockdown or during a period of isolation, unless your lockdown rules allow for medical consultations and treatments.

A patch of hot red skin that looks inflamed and increases in size, often causing a temperature and feeling unwell

Any acute inflammation of the skin or the legs that occurs without an obvious cause such as local trauma, must be thought of as probable infection (cellulitis). This can spread relatively fast and make you feel very unwell. You should consult a doctor straight away as you may well need some antibiotics. Cellulitis can happen without any underlying cause or may be secondary to an underlying problem. However, this can be investigated in time, particularly if the problem recurs.

- **Outside of a lockdown or isolation** - the development of an acutely inflamed patch of skin on the legs, particularly if it starts increasing in size and feels hot, is a medical emergency as it is likely to be in infection that can spread. You should contact your family doctor or emergency department for assessment and treatment.

- **During lockdown or isolation** - the development of an acutely inflamed patch of skin of the legs, particularly if it starts increasing in size and feels hot, is a medical emergency as it is likely to be an infection that can spread. You should contact your family doctor or emergency department for assessment and treatment. As this is an urgent or emergency case, you should do this even if you are in a lockdown or in isolation.

As a final note, I have tried to keep away from merely giving a list of what to do in each situation, as venous disease varies between people, and lockdown rules vary between countries. Currently, in the UK you are able to leave your home in lockdown for any medical appointment or treatment. However, this might change. In other countries, rules might be different.

I hope that by explaining venous disease and treatments more fully, this will help you make a decision about your condition and the urgency that it requires, based on an understanding of what might be going on and what the possible risks are.

I hope that you have found this book useful, and if you have any questions, or suggestions, please contact me through the website www.thewhiteleyclinic.co.uk.

If at any time you feel concerned about your health then it is best to make an appointment with a medical professional. Medical services for venous conditions are still running in some countries at the time of writing; in others you may need to do this by video call or telephone. However, health is of paramount importance and so if you are worried do seek advice. This book is intended to be a helpful guide for you to see what path you could take. However, it cannot hope to give personalised advice and cannot replace a personal consultation with a health care professional. Therefore, if you have any doubt, you should book an appointment with a medical professional.

Previous books by Mark S Whiteley:

Understanding Venous Reflux - the Cause of Varicose Veins and Venous Leg Ulcers
(ISBN: 978-1-908586-00-1)

Leg Ulcer Treatment Revolution
(ISBN: 978-1-908586-05-6)

Pelvic Congestion Syndrome - Chronic Pelvic Pain and Pelvic Venous Disorders
(ISBN: 978-1-908586-07-0)

Edited by Mark S Whiteley:

Advances in Phlebology and Venous Surgery Volume 1
(Paperback: ISBN: 978-1-908586-03-2)
(Hardback: ISBN: 978-1-908586-04-9)

About the Author

Professor Mark S Whiteley is an internationally recognised expert in venous disease including varicose veins, venous leg ulcers and pelvic congestion syndrome.

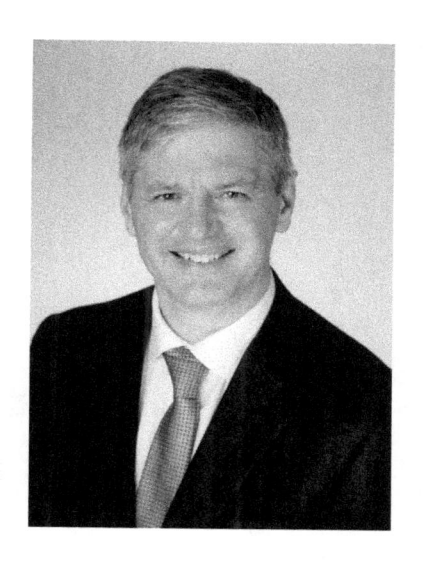

Mark performed the first endovenous surgery for varicose veins in the UK in March 1999, and invented the TRLOP technique to close incompetent perforators in 2001 along with his colleague Judy Holdstock. He set up The Whiteley Clinic as a centre of excellence for venous disorders in 2002, and the College of Phlebology in 2011 to share his knowledge with other healthcare professionals around the world. He performed the first clinical cases of High Intensity Focused Ultrasound (HIFU) for varicose veins in the world in 2019.

Mark has written over a hundred peer-reviewed research papers on venous disease, has won many national and international awards for his research into venous disease and is a regular speaker at international conferences on venous subjects. He became a visiting Prof to the University of Surrey in 2013, sits on the editorial board of the Journal of Vascular Surgery Venous and Lymphatic disorders and also is a reviewer of venous research for many journals.

Mark continues to work to bring new ideas and technology to venous patients, to improve results from venous surgery and to get the best outcomes possible.

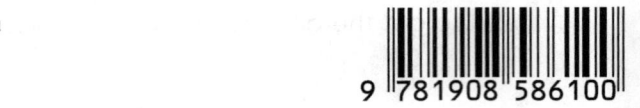

CPSIA information can be obtained
at www.ICGtesting.com
Printed in the USA
BVHW041336300121
599166BV00007B/1389

9 781908 586100